11/12/09

D0814594

SURVIVE CANCER!

"A full and meaningful life must involve some risks or there can be no growth."

—Kathleen Turner

SURVIVE
CANCER!

A Natural Approach to Healing and Prevention

SUSAN MOSS

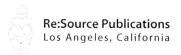

Re:Source Publications
Los Angeles, California

Published in the United States of America by:
Re:Source Publications
4767 York Blvd.
Los Angeles, CA 90042
323-255-3382
www.susanhmoss.com

Publisher's Cataloging-in-Publication
(Provided by Quality Books, Inc.)
    Moss, Susan.
        Survive cancer! : overcoming and preventing cancer
    the natural way / by Susan Moss. -- 1st ed.
        p. cm.
        Includes bibliographical references and index.
        ISBN-13: 978-09642329-2-1
        ISBN-10: 09642329-2-8

        1. Cancer--Alternative treatment. 2. Cancer--
    Prevention. 3. Naturopathy.   I. Title.

    RC271.A62M67 2009   616.99'406
                                 QBI09-600009

Printed in the United States of America

Cover: Susan Moss in her studio
All paintings by Susan Moss
Front Cover Painting: "EarthPeace", oil on canvas, 7 ft. x 6 ft., 2007
Spine Painting: "Earthslide 361", crayon, oil and graphite on hardwood panel,
  8 ft. x 4 ft., 2008
Back Cover Painting: "Ocean Park Peace" (for Richard), oil on canvas,
7 ft. x 5 ft., 2002

Text and cover design: Dotti Albertine

To my father, Ben Moss,
who lived to be 94,
and who taught me that there
are natural ways to get well.

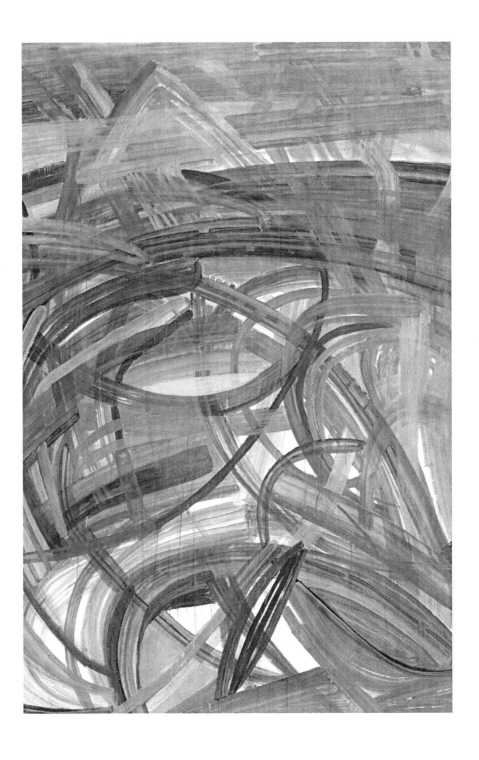

CONTENTS

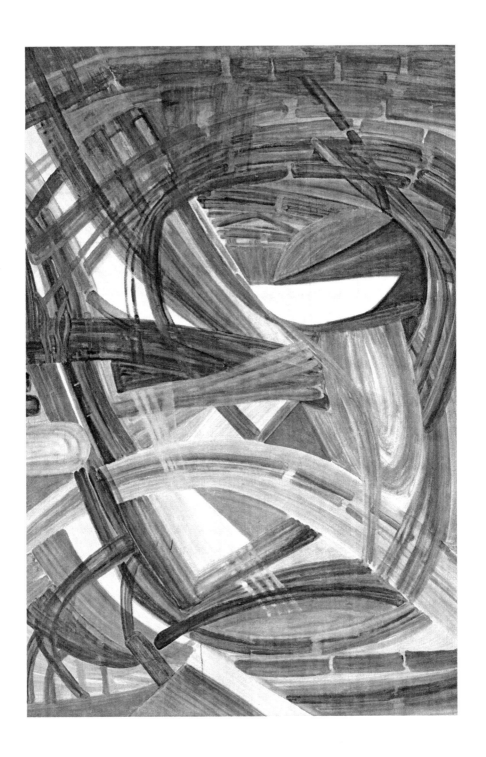

F O R E W O R D

by James R. Privitera, M.D.

I FEEL HONORED to have been asked to write the foreword for Susan Moss' second book. I wrote the foreword for her first book, ***Keep Your Breasts! Preventing Breast Cancer the Natural Way***, that was so beautifully written. I wasn't certain that another book could possibly be as informative and captivating. However, ***Survive Cancer! Overcoming and Preventing Cancer the Natural Way***, once again shows the same passion in the writing of experiences in her own remarkable journey to overcoming and preventing any recurrence of Cancer. It is also a detailed compilation of data to help the reader expand his or her knowledge of Cancer and aid the readers on their own quest for better health. Other inspirational pioneer Cancer survivors' stories are also included.

Because of the importance of her first book, I show a slide of the book cover in my lectures, and I also make the book available to my patients. Over the last thirty years I have treated hundreds of people with Cancer. Many were women with Breast Cancer and I am always proud of those who are willing to seek the information on expanding their understanding of the treatments and modalities that are available.

Susan Moss is one of those people who didn't settle for the standard treatments; instead she set out on her own personal journey, experiencing her amazing victory over breast and uterine Cancer using only Alternative treatments.

Today we find more large medical centers are opening Alternative Medicine departments to meet the public demand for an alternative to the standard drugs, surgery, and radiation. I have often told my patients that what is called "Alternative" should really be the standard, as natural therapies have been around long before any drug companies were built. Can any of us argue with the therapies that naturally support the body to bring it back to full and glowing health without destructive "side effects"? Not me!

Susan's book is not only for people with Cancer, but extremely important for those who are in remission and also for prevention. In fact, any person seeking a healthier and longer life can benefit from this book. I am certain that she will have the gratitude of all who read it.

I am personally grateful that she wrote it.

ACKNOWLEDGMENTS

THANK YOU TO THE Cancer Survivors who pioneered the way to Natural Healing and inspired this book. You will meet them in the forthcoming chapters.

Thank you Dr. James Privitera, Deepak Chopra, Dean Ornish, John Robbins, Nancy Brinker of the Susan B.Koman Foundation, Lorraine Rosenthal of the Cancer Control Society, Dr. Lorraine Day, Suzanne Somers, Dr. Vicki Hufnagel, John Finnegan, Dr.Wayne C Furr, and Meryl Streep who offered much encouragement and endorsements. Thank you Gary Null for participation in the PBS special and putting my story in several of your books. Thank you David J.Hess for allowing my story to be told in your book, *Women Confront Cancer*. Thanks to the Canadians for allowing me to participate and speak at two of their World Conferences on Breast Cancer. I couldn't have gotten the word out without my hard-working PR agent, Irwin Zucker.

My German publisher, Axel Berendes at Flamingos and my Dutch publisher, Judice at Triangel, I owe much gratitude.

No book could have been written and presented to the public without the generous help of my parents Ben and Amy

Moss. Thank you also to encouragement from my niece and nephew, Bridget and Cameron Moss for their enthusiasm.

My friend Robin Quinn and my agent Margret McBride have offered invaluable advice and support. Thank you Marion Philadelphia for her encouragement and help in translating my first book into German. Thank you Petra Bierman, a fine friend, for continually supporting this effort.

To close the curtain, thank you Steve Martin for finding new and original ways to make me laugh through any pain and hardship I've experienced in the last twenty years.

INTRODUCTION

A REVOLUTION in the treatment of Cancer is looming just ahead. We have exhausted ourselves running, walking, fund-rasing and expended endless patience waiting for "them" to find the magic CURE. The paradigm that this fairy-tale wish is based upon is that the handsome Prince of a doctor will save us with his magic sword, cutting out the Cancer and offering his magic potions that will "eradicate" any wicked Cancer cells while also burning them out with magic X-rays. Unfortunately, too often, the "side-effect" of all this gruesome and brutal treatment is the death of the patient.

The theme of this book is the body's amazing ability to heal itself. While it is impossible to cut any disease out of the human body and absurd to assume that poisoning and burning the patient will bring him or her back to good health, the body's own complex healing systems can do the job very well. Cancer is a disease, not just a tumor or cells acting badly. This book is based on the paradigm that Cancer is an immune deficiency disease that can be healed by the body's own defenses we were all inherently born with. We can learn to harness these systems in order to get well. Only the person afflicted with Cancer can do the hard but gratifying and rewarding work that will bring back good health. What is the plan, where is the route one must take? What are the character traits of people who heal themselves, either from scratch or after the medical treatment fails them?

This book offers a program, a guideline for help in regaining health from any Cancer. It offers my story and other people's story who took charge of their disease and found a path back to glowing health.

What strengths did these people find that they had? How did they do it? And what valuable tips can they offer us? You will find many inspirational stories in the following chapters.

MY NATURAL HEALING JOURNEY

Eighteen years ago, in the early nineties, I conquered my own Breast and Uterine Cancer utilizing an all-natural health Program I named MOTEP—Marathon Olympic Tumor Eradication and Prevention Program. I chose to use myself as a Human Guinea Pig to see if the body itself could heal Cancer, if supported by a strong emotional, spiritual, mental, and physical program with lots of good nutrition and exercise. I compiled this program, utilizing my own experience of what I call "Self-Lumpectomy," with additional help from Alternative authors on the subject. Still, to take charge of my ill health alone based mostly on my own theories and experience took a lot of guts. To tell the truth, I was terrified! Yet at the same time, my strong intuition told me that I could do it.

My first experience performing "Self-Lumpectomy" was ridding myself of a lump in my neck in the area where the lymph nodes filter out toxins. In the seventies, I had been using toxic acrylic paints with barrels of Rhoplex for my canvases that sold around the world. I used great quantities of this material which, I was later to learn, is carcinogenic, to produce paintings for large commissions. One public commission was for a quartet of ten-foot paintings for a new hotel tower in downtown Los Angeles, the city where I reside. I completed this commission; at the same time knowing the material was adversely affecting my health. Over many years of using this material, my health slowly declined. By 1979, toward the end of the "Black Forest" series of paintings I dedicated to my Grandparents, Edith and Richard Hecht, I was totally losing my health. Not only had a lump formed in the right side of my neck, but I had trouble breathing, fatigue, and began to lose a lot of weight, seemingly in chunks, off my normally slim body. I looked emaciated.

I had to choose to either stop using this material or continue to become extremely ill. I stopped using Rhoplex and acrylic paint before doing number eighteen of the series. The Hebrew sign for eighteen is the same as "Life"; I chose to live. It was terribly difficult to give up this material that gave me unbelievably beautiful, transparent, yet hard glazes resembling stained glass. It was the perfect painting material, drying overnight so that it could be worked over the next day. I could sand it to get a view through all the transparent layers. The result was spectacular.

One wealthy collector, who had become my patron, told me he loved these paintings so much that he would "buy everything I did with Rhoplex." There were so many reasons I fiercely wanted to continue using this carcinogenic material. I had found the perfect painting medium. Not only did it yield beautiful, durable paintings that sold and thus provided me with an economic base to continue painting, it created Museum interest in my work as well. My career seemed to depend on this incredible, but toxic material.

It was a tortuous decision. I knew I could no longer paint with it.

At UCLA Medical Center, they performed a biopsy. They told me the cells in my lump were "right on the verge of Cancer" and that if I continued using the material, I would develop Cancer. The Doctor also told me that if I did not get rid of the lump in one year, he would operate and take it out.

LEARNING VISUALIZATION

With that deadline, I compiled a simplified health program I did not name. I discovered Visualization from an article in the *L.A. Times* about O. Carl Simonton who found his Cancer patients did well when he taught them to visualize Pac-men eating their Cancer cells and use other imagery they would devise themselves.

The visualization exercise I did every morning consisted of the following steps: first, I would turn on the stereo, finding some loud rock music. I would then visualize a line-up of miniature men in white coats with a large rope. These men would proceed to march down my neck with this strong rope and tie it around the lump in my neck. I would then pull the rope out, with the men and the tumor to the beat of the music. Up and out, I pulled and pulled. I had to pull very hard to get all these men out, their strong rope, and the tumor! I would actually "see" this happening and I would "view" the lump that was pulled out.

I also devised topical, natural treatments, rubbing the lump with a half-cut lemon for the direct application of Vitamin C. Weakened and losing weight rapidly, my health deteriorating to an alarming degree, I talked an architect friend into running on the beach with me. He urged me on, as I was easily fatigued. My Dad, into alternative health before it was trendy, bought me a juicer, and I began to make carrot juice every evening. Along with giving up all paint and turning to crayon drawings, and giving up an emotionally turbulent relationship with a handsome, emotionally disturbed young man, this comprised my total health program. My personal life was gone, my economic base had vanished, my health had deteriorated and my weight was also going down the tubes, as pound after pound left me for outer space! My roommate, who had experience working with Cancer patients, got scared and moved out.

I later read in the newspaper that fifty-five employees of Rohm and Haas, the manufacturer of the barrels of Rhoplex I used, had contracted Cancer. What kept me going? I was terrified yet I steadfastly kept to my schedule: juicing, practicing visualization, running on the beach, and doing crayon drawings—that was my whole life. And yet there was one other characteristic that this yellow-green, toxic, sickly looking, beyond skinny and sinking fast lady had. I had the determination to get well! I had the *tenacity* to stick to this schedule, as I very slowly began to revive, come back to life as I knew it before my system became inundated with toxic materials and weakened by emotional turmoil.

REGAINING HEALTH

Health came back very slowly. But persistence paid off! My health very slowly, but steadily, returned. Within the year allotted to me by the Doctor, I was rid of the lump in my neck to his complete astonishment. He was expecting and ready to perform surgery.

I had learned this crucial fact: when the body is detoxified and de-stressed, when the immune system is supported with good nutrition and exercise, supportive relationships, and *the will to live*, health will begin slowly, but surely, returning. When the body reaches a certain stage of health, it will discard the tumor as unneeded, often in a most dramatic performance! Thus I had learned "Self-Lumpectomy," that is getting rid of lumps in the body without invasive surgery or any Medical treatments other than diagnosis. After this "self-lumpectomy," I was able to rebuild my health, slowly regaining my proper weight.

After a year of doing large-scale crayon drawings, I was asked to show the work at the Albright-Knox Gallery in Buffalo, New York. This is one of the foremost museums in the country. The show was a success, and after selling five drawings, I rented a car to tour the East and Toronto, Canada. In Toronto I met a new man, Mark, who was emotionally healthy. We had a wonderful time together. I thoroughly enjoyed my regained well-being. I felt fortunate and blessed.

ANOTHER BOUT WITH TUMORS

For the next eight or nine years, I took better care of my physical health. I switched to oil paints, discovering how to use non-toxic linseed oil made by a health-food company in Canada to make mediums, and using Citrus-based thinners instead of strong turpentine or mineral spirits to thin my paints and clean my brushes. Slowly, my collectors came around to my new techniques and began acquiring the oils. By 1988, I was again prospering. However, in 1989, a recession hit the country and I was unable to sell my art. As a result, I became depressed and again neglected to take care of myself. I also found myself, once again, attracted to a man who was not loyal to me. He often talked about his other girlfriends and even his ex-wife whom he still visited. Finally he decided to marry the girlfriend who had waited twenty years for him to commit to her The resulting emotional turmoil combined with the financial tension began, once again, taking a big toll on my health, although I was too depressed to pay much attention.

By December 1990, I once again found my health jeopardized. My gynecologist, on a routine check-up, found a tumor in my left breast and one in my uterus. He diagnosed me with Breast and Uterine Cancer and told me in no uncertain terms to see a surgeon.

I said "No."

He repeatedly called me at the studio, insisting that I see a surgeon, in no uncertain terms, in a most forceful way.

I gave him the same answer over the phone. "No."

After several tries, he finally relented enough to tell me to come back for another check-up in two months. It was then that I developed my formal program that I called "MOTEP."

When the doctor found the tumors, a wake-up call was issued to my depressed trance. Reality startled me into awareness. I decided, then and there, that I was willing to do ANYTHING to regain my health.

DECIDING TO GET WELL

I first decided *I wanted to get well.* This is the crucial first step. Decide why you want to get well and the body will begin its healing journey right then and there!

Devising and then going on my own program, MOTEP was the next step to start to reverse my deteriorating health. I was able to begin to fight for and slowly, but surely, to rebuild my health. To my doctor's astonishment, I was rid of both tumors within the "deadline" he had given me— only two months! To him, this was just a "watch and wait" period, and would only result in him having to straightjacket me, if necessary, to get me to the surgeon! He had no idea that "self-lumpectomy" was a viable option. And why should he? The Medical Establishment considers "spontaneous remission" of tumors and Cancer a freak occurrence. Certainly, tumors and Cancer that disappear without medical treatment are considered rare and magical, an event that would be entered in "Ripley's Believe it or Not!" Definitely, they would never think of recommending this to a patient!

My Doctor, however, was open-minded enough to urge me to share my information with others. He suggested a video. First, however, I decided to write a book. During the next seven months it took me to rebuild my health back to normal, I also began to write, *Keep Your Breasts! Preventing Breast Cancer the Natural Way* describing my healing from Breast and Uterine Cancer.

THE TUMOR IS NOT THE DISEASE

I kept up my MOTEP program while writing, as I found that ridding one's body of tumors was not the whole health story. The tumors are only a symptom of a mind-body disease, *not the disease itself.* This is very important because it is a medical misconception that must be cleared up before any progress can be made against this dreaded disease. Cancer is not only about Cancer cells that form a tumor, but also about a weakened, debilitated, toxic body condition and depressed emotional state that allowed these cells to grow and begin to take over. Even after the tumors disappear or are surgically removed, one has to patiently and persistently work to rebuild one's health back to normal. If this is not attended to, the Cancer may return. This leads to the Medical Establishment's use of the terms "remission and recurrence" instead of healed or "cured."

THE MOTEP PROGRAM CAN HELP YOU

Over the last eight years, many Cancer patients have benefited from my program. Many women with suspicious Mammograms have been able to change the results from problem to clear in an astonishingly short time: only ten-days- to-four months. People all over the world have recovered their health using my MOTEP program with or without any Medical treatment. A woman with Stage IV Cancer, considered the last stage, with not just Breast, but also Colon, and Lung Cancer was "supposed to die" within three months even with extensive surgery including the removal of her breast, one of her lungs and part of her colon thus needing a colostomy bag.

She said, "No, thank you," got my book from the bookstore and called me. Fourteen years later she is fully alive, working and traveling. The Doctors are incredulous. Her story will be included in this volume.

My first book has been, from the first printing, in all the

bookstores and many libraries and has been translated into German and Dutch. It seemed time to write another book for anyone fighting *any* Cancer or with the prescient curiosity to want to try to prevent it. This book is especially important to people in "remission," those who do not want to experience a recurrence. I believe the MOTEP program that so helped me and so many others worldwide, can benefit anyone facing any form of Cancer. It is my hope that this book will benefit and inspire you, your relatives, friends and co-workers and anyone whose health you care about. The life you save may be your own!

CHAPTER 1

Staying Alive—The Will to Live

A DIAGNOSIS OF CANCER is the most terrifying news anyone can receive about the state of his or her health. Yet 1.4 million of us in the U.S. will receive this horrifying report this year. Worldwide there are ten million Cancer cases diagnosed yearly, and six million deaths from Cancer. The American Cancer Society estimates that every twenty-five minutes someone is diagnosed with Cancer in the U.S. As treatment now stands, fifty-to-sixty percent of people contracting Cancer will die within five years of their diagnosis. Over ten thousand Americans die each week of Cancer—fifteen hundred a day! I don't believe this is necessary. I don't believe Cancer has to be a "terminal" disease.

YOU CAN LIVE THROUGH CANCER

It is a proven fact that you can live through Cancer. The body itself is well equipped to deal with this disease.

This book is different than others you might find because it is based on empowerment of the ill person, and discusses natural means of getting well. In other words, your health is all in your own hands. Does this surprise you?

It is my personal opinion, after attending too many funerals, that Medical Treatments for Cancer, which have essentially remained unchanged in fifty years, are archaic and outmoded. Chemotherapy is often ineffective, destructive, and temporary in reducing Cancer cells, and radiotherapy is only temporarily effective, and often even more destructive. In fact, radiation is carcinogenic, causing more Cancer down the line.

According to "Cancer Treatment Reviews", June 2001,[1] the majority of Prostate Cancer patients relapse within two-to-three years after the initiation of treatment. There is a high mortality rate in Prostate Cancer because of bone metastases. Of the ten million worldwide cases, the World Health Organization states that only one-third can be effectively treated. In a review of Breast Cancer patients treated with chemotherapy and radiation, reported in *Breast Cancer Research and Treatment*, July 16, 2002,[2] showed that evidence from two randomized clinical trials of radiation following chemotherapy, whether delayed or not showed no impact on either local or distant control of the disease or survival.

Medical Treatments for Cancer have become a multi-billion dollar enterprise, a gigantic machinery, disconnected from the purpose of healing sick people. This profit-driven industry, a dinosaur of greed and billion-dollar profits, will soon, I predict, die out as the understanding of Cancer expands from its primitive, barbaric stage into the realm of enlightened, Mind-body, "Alternative" medicine. We are presently witnessing an amazing Consumer-driven overhaul

1 Homby, F.E., " Prognostic and Predictive Factors in Prostate Cancer" Cancer Treatment Reviews, Vol. 27, #3, June 2001
2 "Delay in Adjuvant Radiation Treatment and Outcomes in Breast Cancer"

of Modern Medicine and a drastic turn-around to Alternative Therapies, information and products, by the very people affected by Cancer. For instance, eighty percent of Breast Cancer patients now incorporate alternative therapies into their treatment regimens.

THREE STEPS TO GETTING WELL

From my experience, there are essentially three steps anyone with any form of Cancer must go through to get well. In my opinion they are not surgery, chemotherapy, and radiation, treatments that debilitate the body and usually are only a temporary "solution." They are:

1. Detoxifying the body
2. De-stressing the mind
3. Bolstering the Will to Live

This chapter addresses the most important of these three, the basis for all good health: *The Will to Live.* Without this core of strength, no amount of Medical Treatment or Alternative Treatments can succeed either alone or in combination. So let's look at the disease we may be facing.

WHAT IS CANCER?

Cancer is a cellular disorder. Normally cells divide in an orderly way. They do their job in replicating the tissue they coincide with such as skin tissue, breast tissue, or colon tissue, whatever tissue it is their job to replicate. This job is accomplished through messengers: molecules called hormones, growth factors, and cytokines (cells that move). The cells actually communicate with each other as well as with the brain through neurotransmitters—neuro-receptors and neuro-receivers. They are polite and have a tail that has a sensor to alert them to other oncoming cells that they politely go around. They are orderly.

Suddenly, in the disease we call Cancer, cells multiply without control, wildly only reproducing themselves. Cancer cells are deformed, immature, rude, selfish, asocial cells that use the nutrition of other cells, rampage over normal cells, and franchise themselves out, metastasizing to other parts of the body in their single-minded goal of destruction.

Instead of replicating local tissue, they form their own tumor or "neoplasm" (new growth) that the healthy body normally has no need for. A protein coating is then formed over the Cancer cells to cordon them off to protect the body from these malignant, damaged cells. However, this tumor soon sets up a life of its own, creating its own blood supply to feed itself regardless of the body's needs. If it is able to proceed, it will soon erode the energy of the host and use up the nutrition of the healthy cells, leaving the person emaciated. Patients often die of Cachexia, or wasting away. The patient's normal cells have been robbed of the nutrition they need. Cancer cells are parasitical users, intent on a selfish mission of destruction, and are only "looking out for number one." They are sneaky, underhanded robbers of life.

Medical treatment currently focuses on cutting out and destroying these cells. But too often they only return leading to the terms "remission" and "recurrence." "Cure-rate" is a misleading term used to sell Cancer treatments. There is no outside "cure" for Cancer. Only the body itself can heal it.

CANCER CANNOT BE CUT OUT OF THE BODY

Can Measles, Mumps, Chicken pox lumps, the Flu, Colds, Arthritis or any other disease be cut out of the body? The answer, of course, is no. *No disease can be cut out of the body.* Cancer is a whole-body-mind-spirit illness, but because it often forms a tumor, the prevailing modus operandi is to cut out the tumor calling it a "local" disease according to where that tumor was found. But the tumor is only one symptom of a whole-body, mind, and soul degeneration. The tumor is only a messenger. The message it announces is that the whole person is extremely ill, not just in that one specific area. In my opinion and most Alternative Healers, Cancer is NEVER a "localized disease." When health is rebuilt, the body will have no more use for a tumor, and the immune and healing systems will destroy it, sometimes in a most dramatic manner. But Cancer is not considered in light of a person's illness by mainstream medicine. It is looked upon as a tumor or an abnormally high white-blood cell count, an enemy that has to be mechanically cut out, destroyed with toxic drugs, or zapped with dangerous, carcinogenic radiation! *But Cancer can only happen when an individual's total health has deteriorated.* We are not robots with a tumor. Take it out and we are robots without a tumor? We are not robots; we are desperately ill people. The tumor is only one important clue, a symptom, for our extremely deteriorated health. It is a messenger bringing to us this very urgent warning: "You can't keep destroying this body or you will lose it."

WHY DO WE GET CANCER?

Why does a person get Cancer? The cells are only a reflection of our Life Condition. WE ARE OUR CELLS. Our cells become chaotic and out-of-control when our lives are chaotic and out-of-control. If you are working with carcinogenic materials, the Will to Live must be strong enough for you to find other materials to work with, or another job that does not endanger your life. If you live around nuclear radiation, the Will to Live must motivate you to move. If you are in emotional turmoil, the Will to Live will help you give up or turn around the relationship that is making you miserable. If you have experienced a major emotional loss in your life, the Will to Live will guide you to seek therapy or counseling to help you through your grief. If you have given up your dreams in order to sacrifice your life to others, it's time to begin a new life, one directed toward fulfilling your life-long ambitions. If you have gotten out-of-shape and overweight, the Will to Live will help you to choose organic fruits, vegetables and whole grains, beans, fish, nuts and seeds for your meals. It will further induce you to join a gym or incorporate one into your home, start a walking program with neighbors or on your own, and get into marvelous shape.

EXPERIMENTS TO INJECT CANCER CELLS
INTO A HEALTHY PERSON COMPLETELY FAIL

When health is restored, Cancer will NATURALLY disappear. Cancer cells abhor and will die in a happy, clean, oxygenated, vitamin enriched environment. They thrive in a sluggish, fat-and sugar filled, alcohol and tobacco laden, drug-filled, overweight, toxic, depressed, distressed and frustrated body/mind condition.

As an example of this, it was shown by Nobel Prize winner Otto Warburg that normal cells deprived of Oxygen could become Cancer cells. Cancer cells multiply by fermentation using glucose (sugar), while healthy cells use Oxygen. Simply put, eating lots of fats and sweets and sitting around a lot encourages Cancer, while doing plenty of exercise and going off sugar, meat, and dairy products, discourages it. When people worked on a farm, doing hard, physical labor, and ate fresh fruits and vegetables without a lot of chemical pesticides, Cancer rates were very low.

Is it a surprise then that anorexic women have a low Breast Cancer rate? While I am not recommending starvation, calorie restriction and keeping slender has proven Cancer prevention powers.

Here is another Classic Maxim:
HAPPY PEOPLE DON'T GET CANCER.

When I lecture on Cancer, I ask, "Does the Doctor upon finding a tumor in your body ask, 'Are you happy?'"

This always gets a laugh. The Doctor most likely will say the same exact thing my Doctor said to me, only three little words, "See a surgeon!" He is not concerned with your emotional state or your stress level, or any of your lifestyle problems. He will not suggest a career change, a divorce, group therapy, or even exercise or weight loss. He will not ask you how you are sleeping or *if* you are sleeping.

He will, most likely, strongly urge mechanical procedures: cutting the tumor out, burning with radiation, and poisoning you with Chemotherapy drugs. In contrast, in other older and wiser cultures such as India and China, the whole person is considered, not just the symptoms of disease. The ancients believed that dream interpretation should be included in Cancer treatment. What is the disease trying to tell you about your life?

ROSEMARY CLOONEY'S CANCER

In the *Los Angeles Times* it was reported that "Rosemary Clooney's publicist has confirmed that the seventy-four year old singer's Cancer has returned. She was said to be in serious condition, undergoing treatment at home. Doctors at Minnesota's Mayo Clinic removed the upper lobe of Clooney's left lung in January (reported in the June 28, 2002 issue)."The surgery was considered successful."

"We got it all." Isn't that what they say?

However, the next day she died of Cancer.

Why is surgery considered a treatment for a disease? What illness can be cut out of the body?

That wonderful songbird I loved to listen to as a teen-ager—Rosemary Clooney. Let's look at her life. Obituaries can teach us a lot about Cancer. The seeds of Cancer may actually start an unhappy childhood that many creative people have experienced. Rosemary's parents separated frequently. Her father was a heavy drinker and rarely around. Clooney and her siblings were farmed out to various relatives.

We see that she grew up surrounded by the insecurity of emotional turmoil and not knowing with whom or where she would live next. This may have affected her Will to Live. However, like many who shine in life as bright as stars, she compensated for this miserable childhood with her voice and singing talents. She used her vocal talents as a form of therapy.

However, she repeated this pattern of emotionally disruptive family relationships when she married Jose Ferrar, had five children with him, and then divorced him. That same year she remarried him. Then six years later she divorced him again. He was continually unfaithful to her.

When her friend Robert F. Kennedy was assassinated, she was staying at the hotel. During a subsequent engagement in Reno, she broke down, walked off the stage and took a dangerous drive. On a two-lane mountain highway, she drove on the wrong side of the road, playing a form of Russian roulette with oncoming cars and saying, "That's one for you God," as she barely missed hitting them.

Cells cannot function in a healthy, normal fashion when their environment is emotional chaos, and the brain in sending signals that indicate a "death wish." They will mirror this turmoil. **Our cells are us. We are our cells.**

DO YOU WANT TO LIVE?

Whenever someone calls me or approaches me about Cancer, the first thing I ask them is, "Do you want to live?" If there is ambivalence in their hesitation, I know their Will to Live is not strong.

This question is not self-evident. It is extremely pertinent because even though they called me, an unconscious wish to die may have been present for some time, perhaps years.

The second question I ask is, "Have you had a major stress in the last year-and-a-half to two years or more?" Or I might even be so bold as to add, "When do you think your Cancer started?"

Over the fourteen years that I have asked this question, I have never failed to get a swift reply.

John, an entertainment writer, walked into the art gallery where I was viewing paintings with a well-bandaged hand. When I asked him what happened, he told me he had just undergone an operation for Skin Cancer. They had taken off quite a large section of skin.

"What happened to you two years ago?" I asked. I had never met John in my life yet I knew he would have an answer.

"My Dad died," he said without a moment's hesitation.

I explained to him how the white blood cells that patrol the body looking for Cancer cells to destroy actually stop moving when a person is deeply depressed. This can be seen under a microscope.

Without this patrol, the Cancer cells we all carry in our body, which are usually caught by the white blood cells and destroyed, have free reign to multiply unchecked.

I also talked to him about his diet and exercise habits. He said he liked to eat pastries and didn't exercise. When I told him that Cancer cells replicate by fermentation using glucose (sugar) instead of oxygen that the normal cells use that exercise would supply, he began to understand his Cancer. Would he give up eating pastries regularly? Would he incorporate an exercise program? Perhaps this new knowledge will help him to understand his Skin Cancer—how his own behavior contributed to it. Cutting out the Cancer might work temporarily. However, no permanent "cure" will happen until he changes his habits and his body begins the healing process. He has to discover the *cause*. Without this investigation and fundamental life-change, odds are the Cancer may grow back.

YOU DETERMINE YOUR HEALTH

When you review your life and begin to understand how you have participated in your deteriorating health, it is easier to reclaim it. And it **can** be reclaimed, but not usually without vigorous effort or vigilant change. Your health can be rebuilt. If you are willing to do the work, incorporating new, healthy habits and taking a hard look at the direction of your life, you will see the results. When I was diagnosed with Breast and Uterine Cancer, I made the determination that I was willing to do *anything* in order to reclaim my health!

You can return to full health. But a diet, exercise, mental and spiritual program will only help if the Will to Live is strong.

Here is another noteworthy obituary. The headline is "Silas Trim Bissell, Age sixty; Spent Years as a Fugitive After Bombing Attempt." He died of Brain Cancer.

Silas inherited a carpet-cleaning fortune but chose to live a life of destruction at war with his environment. He was an award-winning poet, and a tenure-track professor who gave up his teaching job and began a life as a Radical with his wife. The "Weatherman" was a group he joined to protest the Viet Nam War. He and his wife placed a paper bag containing a homemade bomb on the steps of the ROTC building at the University of Washington. The explosive failed to go off. However, the marriage bombed! After the divorce, Silas' wife was apprehended and spent three years in jail.

Alone and on the run, Bissell was desperately unhappy. He moved anonymously from city to city, walking for miles every day because "I did not know what to do with myself."

Finally he moved to Eugene, Oregon where he managed to build a new life as a Nurse's aid and went back to school to learn physical therapy. However, the FBI caught up with him after seventeen years and arrested him on evidence from one of his friends who betrayed him. Silas served seventeen months in jail. He was diagnosed with Brain Cancer four years after his release. How did his lifestyle, his everyday War with his environment, contribute to his disease? Cells cannot exist peacefully within our body when we are constantly at war with our surroundings. They are only a reflection of ourselves. They are mirrors of how we treat ourselves and others. When we are in a constant state of turmoil, our cells will be chaotic, leading to Dis-Ease.

ANOTHER LIFE CUT SHORT

Here is another life cut short: Daniel Case III, age forty-four, who fueled the Wall Street Internet boom. A photo shows a very handsome, robust, extremely vigorous looking man, who spent more than twenty years putting his heart into the building up, financing and investing of computer companies. Case became one of the most influential bankers during the bull market decade in the nineties. He was an important part of the youth-driven Internet boom. But his efforts and company were taken over by Chase in 1999, when many of these companies began to bottom out and fail. Although Chase made him the head of this division, two years later, he stepped down from his day-to-day responsibilities after he was diagnosed with Brain Cancer.

Was the distress of losing his battle to maintain the company he had put his heart and soul into building up over two decades, a major factor in his losing his health?

LOOK FOR CAUSES OF CANCER IN YOUR LIFE

I believe in looking for causes for Cancer and clues from these obituaries and the interviews I have done over the past fifteen years with people with Cancer. They always point to distress as one of the major factors.

A group of people with Cancer ranging from problem mammograms to stage four Cancer met in my studio every Wednesday evening. It was surprising to me that the worst case, the stage four Cancer that Orlan had with a survival expectation of only three months with extensive surgery, turned out to be a long-term, fourteen year, so far and still working, survival story with NO surgery. Five of her close relatives had died within two years including her Mother whom she was taking care of. She subsequently developed Breast, Colon, and Lung Cancer. Her Doctors advised her to remove a breast, part of her colon and one of her lungs. She would have to carry a Colostomy bag. She then could live for three more months! Her quality of life, during that short period, would be close to zero.

She said "No thank you", went to the bookstore and discovered my book on self-healing.

With no surgery, but with a strong Will to Live, Orlan not only took responsibility for her own health, she helped everyone in the group. She not only followed my MOTEP program, but also read everything she could about what she could do for herself Alternatively. Her strong Will to Live was reflected in her voice that reverberated with determination. Her force of will helped her to change her diet. She had relied on fast foods such as French fries and Cokes. Changing to vegetables, fruits, and whole grains, adding exercise, participating in our group, helping others, communicating her feelings, and doing things she always wanted to do, such as travel, but had put off because of her self-sacrifice in caring for her sick Mother, has paid off in astounding longevity. Her Doctors are stunned! Without any Medical treatment other than diagnosis, this Stage IV Cancer "victim" is alive and working!

THE WILL TO LIVE WILL HELP YOU TO SURVIVE

The Will to Live involves tapping our inner strength. It means finding and appreciating the gift of life we have been given. It needs reasons to live. It needs *appreciation* for the wonderful things we have in our life. It means having hope that tomorrow will bring us what we want and need. It requires us to visualize a happy life, giving us the rich rewards and pleasures that are there for the taking if only we have the courage to pluck them. It requires that we get back up from our failures and defeats, and try again in a new or modified direction. It means tackling obstacles, emotional difficulties, failed relationships and financial defeats, with new ideas, new energy, new relationships or renewing old ones on a new path of love. It means going back home after the funeral of a loved one with enriched memories instead of only feelings of loss and futility. It means finding new materials to work with or moving to a healthier environment. It means expressing your feelings, standing up for yourself, expressing your needs and wants, and especially, finding the ability to get angry when necessary. It means accepting responsibility, opening up, moving on, finding new avenues for your talents, maturing and growing. It means finding hope for the future and finding the motivation to live it. This all takes tremendous courage.

In England in 1972, Researcher Steven Greer and his colleagues investigated characteristics of Cancer patients and how they accepted their diagnosis compared with their outcomes. He grouped people into four categories:

1. *Fighting Spirit*: These people accepted their diagnosis but saw a challenge that they would bring optimism to get them through it. They sought out information and began to actively get involved in treatment decisions. They saw a problem that would be solved and took up the challenge. Natural fighters, they were highly motivated and immediately got involved in every way they could.

2. *Denial*: These people refused to accept their diagnosis or minimized its threat. They didn't want to talk or even think about their disease. Yet they were positive and not unaware; they simply didn't wallow in self-pity and knew they would get through whatever faced them.

3. *Stoic acceptance*: These patients accepted their diagnosis, but didn't want to know any more about their disease. They were resigned to whatever fate handed them. They either didn't believe there was anything they could do for themselves or they refused to do anything to help themselves. They were used to bad news and greeted it with silence and a belief in endurance. They didn't complain or ask questions, but stoically accepted their fate.

4. *Helplessness, hopelessness:* These people were
   overwhelmed by their diagnosis. Their lives were
   disrupted and they were anxious and fearful.
   They were exhausted. Worried and panicked, they
   thought in circles. They felt they could control
   nothing in their lives including their actions and
   needs. They took on the role of helpless, hopeless
   victim.

Greer followed these groups of people for fifteen years.
Those who were able to regain their health and remain
recurrence-free were significantly more in the fighting-
spirit or denial groups. These people fared much better than
those with either the stoic acceptance or the helplessness/
hopelessness attitude. After fifteen years, forty-five percent
of the fighters and deniers were alive compared to seventeen percent of more negative, "give-in" or "endure misery"
attitudes.

PASSIVE PATIENTS DO THE WORST

Here is a Classic Maxim in the Medical literature:
PASSIVE PATIENTS FARE THE WORST.

Bolster the Will to Live through your own decisions and
you immediately activate your immune and healing systems
that will hear the message loud and clear. Now is the time
to take charge!

Now take a clean sheet of paper and a pen and answer
these questions as honestly as you can:

- *Do you want to live?* Now write down ten reasons you want to continue your life. Start with the phrase, "I'm lucky I have…" and fill in each blank.

- *Are you willing to do anything, change your life in any way, in order to get well and/or stay well?* List any self-destructive habits you might have such as smoking, drinking, drug addiction, junk food diet, overeating, overweight, high animal fat diet, sugar addiction, repressing your anger, continual conflicts with others, being selfish, being rude, harboring resentment, holding grudges, being stuck in some areas of your life, not living your purpose in life, etc.

- *What image would you draw to sum up your current life-condition?* For instance, if you are a fighter, by nature, you could draw a lion. Have some fun with this one.

- If you have been grieving over lost relationships or lost love ones, write ways you can taper off the grieving process and get on with your life. How can you regain your happiness, perhaps by increasing your social activity, taking a trip, making new friends, helping others?

If you have been diagnosed with Cancer, it is time to heal. If you took the time to answer this questionnaire, you already have taken the first step back to health.

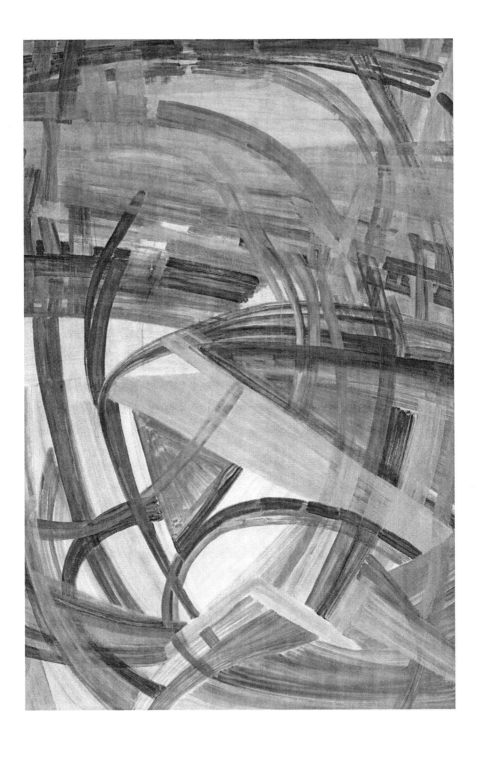

CHAPTER 2

Overcoming the Causes of Cancer

IN HIS BOOK *Speak from the Heart*, Steve Adubato Ph.D. quotes Dr. Elisa Santora, an oncology surgeon and founder and owner of The Breast Care Treatment Center in Livingston, New Jersey. Santora says, "I have spent eighteen years at the bedside of people newly diagnosed with Cancer, being treated, and dying, and they taught me that what they wanted was inner peace. The 'cure' was not the issue—it's the whole person that wants to be healed."

To me, "cure" is a fund-raising, fantasy word. No cure exists for the common cold, yet we can get well. Few people die of the common cold, because after a few days of rest and drinking a lot of liquids, the body successfully fights it off. Although it takes longer and involves more effort, this should be the same, I believe, for Cancer. We may spend billions trying to find an elusive Cure for Cancer, while what we really are looking for is ways to get well again, to support our body in its own heroic efforts to heal our disease. **The magic bullet we are looking for resides within ourselves.**

A new paradigm for Cancer needs to evolve. Destruction of Cancer cells instituted in a war-like, toxic and mutilating fashion while the elusive "cure" is searched for in the

laboratory by a scientist in a white coat looking into a microscope, needs to be replaced by learning the causes of Cancer
and how to overcome them, heal the body, and continue
building health in a natural, nurturing way.

KNOWN CAUSES OF CANCER

So let's go over some of the causes of Cancer that we have
pinpointed to date:

1. **Smoking**: The World Health Organization's sur-
    vey links deaths in the industrialized countries
    to cigarette smoking at a rate of 1.8 million per
    year. According to the American Cancer Society,
    tobacco is the single largest preventable cause of
    Cancer. Tobacco smoke is a much deadlier car-
    cinogen and triggers a broader variety of Cancers
    than researchers had previously believed accord-
    ing to the most comprehensive study of smoking
    ever undertaken. The new study firmly links
    smoking to stomach, liver, cervical, and kidney
    Cancer as well to myeloid leukemia.

    A study of Breast Cancer and how it increases
    with number of years of smoking was reported in
    the August 9, 2002 issue of the *British Medical
    Journal*. According to researchers at the Albert
    Einstein College of Medicine in Bronx, New
    York, women who smoked forty years or longer
    increased their risk of Breast Cancer by sixty
    percent compared to women who never smoked.
    If they used twenty cigarettes or more a day, the
    risk increased eighty-three percent.

A United Nations team examined more than three thousand studies involving millions of smokers. (Reported in *L.A Times*, June 20, 2002.) Smoking destroys the self-cleaning mechanisms of the lungs, paralyzing the small cilia that clean them. This paralysis is the major cause of Lung Cancer. Cigarettes contain one hundred fifty known carcinogens including tar. Carbon monoxide produced in cigarette smoke robs the cells of oxygen. As we have already discussed, Cancer cells thrive in an oxygen-deprived environment.

The Medical System sees Lung Cancer as incurable, using surgery, radiation, and chemotherapy to sometimes postpone death for six months to a year while destroying the quality of life for the patient. Yet Orlan, my star student, has lived on for over fourteen years, despite her Lung, Colon, and Breast Cancer. Still Lung Cancer is one of the hardest to fight. I hope this and other information will help you give up this destructive habit if you smoke.

2. **Abuse of Alcohol and Drugs**: Alcohol is positively associated with a Cancer of the skin called Melanoma, considered a deadly Cancer. For Breast Cancer, the association was highest with women who drank one glass of beer daily, and lowest for women who drank one glass of wine daily. In a study of 90,000 nurses, excess risks often were apparent in low levels of consumption—three to nine glasses a week. ("Cancer

Research" April 1, 1992). In African-American women, one alcoholic drink per week was associated with a 2.7% increased risk of death.[1]

Drugs suppress the immune system. The body is well equipped to deal with disease and infection without added chemicals. We need a strong immune system to fight off Cancer. Why take chances?

3. **Excess Fats in the Diet:** High-fat diets, especially saturated fats from meat and dairy products, promote the growth of mammary tumors in laboratory animals. An ancient Indian seven-volume medical reference, some four thousand years old, lists the cause of Cancer as "overeating dairy foods." Countries with low-fat diets such as Japan, Singapore, and Romania have the lowest Cancer rates. Japan leads with one-eighth the Breast Cancer rate when the Oriental diet is consumed. Soy is substituted for dairy products in Oriental cultures. Countries with the highest fat diets have the biggest Cancer rate: the U.S., Great Britain, and the Netherlands.

4. **Overweight (even the usual five pounds)** The Cable News Network reports in 2002 that the American Institute of Cancer Research Study sought to see how much Americans knew about this link. Although most people knew about overweight and its connection to heart disease and diabetes, only 25% knew about the Cancer risk. "Gaining half a pound per year or five pounds

---

1 "Cancer Causes and Control" July 15, 2002

per decade can contribute to Cancer risk," said Dr. George Bray, professor of medicine at Louisiana State University Medical Center. Sixty-one percent of Americans are either overweight or obese, according to 2002 reports from the Center for Disease Control and prevention. Risks for postmenopausal Breast Cancer, Colon Cancer, Prostate, Esophageal, Endometrial and Kidney Cancer increase among non-smoking, overweight and obese adults according to this report. "It's gaining weight over a long period of time that causes health problems," Bray said.

5. **Refined white flour, sugar, and their products:** Consuming empty calories in foods that have been stripped of all nutritional value can lead to nutritional deficiencies. Vitamin deficiencies have been linked to various Cancers such as Beta- carotene in Breast Cancer. Other vitamins especially important which are linked to Cancer by important scientists such as Linus Pauling and Ernest Krebs include: Vitamin A in the form of Beta-Carotene, The B Vitamins, especially Vitamin B-17, Vitamin C, Vitamin D, and Vitamin E. These vitamins, available in vegetables, fruits, flaxseed and olive oil, and the seeds and kernels of various fruits such as apricots and apples, are stripped in processed foods or thrown or bred out as in seedless varieties of fruits. Eating whole, organic foods has been associated with Cancer

healing. Adding seeds and nuts to our dishes will increase our arsenal of Cancer preventing vitamins.

6. **Caffeine (chocolate, coffee, cola):** Caffeine has been found by researchers at Occidental College to damage the repair mechanisms of the DNA. It also damages the immune system, according to the late nutritionist, John Finnegan. When I called the Breast Center in Van Nuys, California, the one substance they could point to as damaging to the breasts, causing cysts and influencing Breast Cancer, was caffeine.

7. **Birth Control Pills:** Hormonal pills alter the delicate balance of the endocrine system. In order to create the headline, *"Study Debunks Added Cancer Risk with the Pill,"* (*Los Angeles Times,* June 24, 2002), the journalist had to save the last paragraphs for the most important information.

   "The sole exception to the findings (young women who don't smoke showed no increased risks) was women between the ages of 45-64. These women who are taking the pill to alleviate symptoms of menopause, or 'reduce their risk' of Ovarian, and Endometrial Cancer, and benign Breast disease, showed an increased risk of Breast Cancer." In other words, birth control pills seemingly did not affect the Breast Cancer risk of younger woman, most who do not get Breast Cancer, but did affect the woman most at risk (ages

45-64), which is the general age when Breast Cancer strikes.

My earlier research indicated a fourfold increase in Breast Cancer in young women due to birth-control pills according to Pike, et al. 1981-83.[2] Hormone related Cancers account for more than forty percent of all newly diagnosed female Cancers in the United States according to Malcolm C. Pike, noted researcher in the field.

8. **Estrogen Replacement and Hormone-Replacement Therapy:** Back in 1991, *The Los Angeles Times*, April 17, reported that estrogen-replacement therapy caused nearly five thousand cases of Breast Cancer per year. In July 2002, it reported an NIH study of sixteen thousand women was halted when it found a whopping 80 percent increase in Ovarian Cancer for women using it for ten years, and 220 percent in women using HRT for twenty years. The Women's Health Initiative study was halted when it found an increased risk of Breast Cancer, heart attacks, blood clots in legs and lungs, and strokes. All these "side effects" can be fatal. The "gold standard" was a pill derived from pregnant mare's urine, called Premarin. Horses are kept in stalls continually pregnant to derive this "estrogen." The stalls are so small they cannot lie down or move around. It is a cruelty to horses and an insult to women that they need as much estrogen

2 Pike, M.C; Chilvers, C. "Oral Contraceptives and Breast Cancer: the Current Controversy" Journal of the Royal Society of Health, 1985: 1:

as a pregnant horse! Menopausal women are producing less estrogen for a reason; they no longer need it to reproduce. The ovaries still produce some estrogen after menopause, so we are never completely deprived unless they have been surgically removed. You wouldn't drink horse urine, why take it in a pill? Phytoestrogens are called "bio-available" because the body can actually use them, and include soy, cucumbers, black cohosh, ginseng, and dong quai, and phytosterols as in string beans and sweet potatoes. These foods and herbs plus my exercise program, got me through menopause without one hot flash or night sweat. Using natural plants that the body can assimilate protects us, while synthetic drugs from chemicals or animal waste products that toxify and confuse the body can make us ill.

9. **DES:** This synthetic estrogenic hormone (Diestillbestrol) was invented in 1938. Tested in mice, it was found to cause Breast Cancer. Nevertheless, like many drugs actually known to be hazardous to health, it was sent out to the marketplace where it caused considerable and terrible damage. Doctors prescribed the drug to pregnant women to be used as a "preventative" for possible miscarriage. These women sometimes developed Breast Cancer and their yet unborn daughters might later develop Vaginal Cancer as well as being born with deformed genital organs.

   Despite the horrific effects of this synthetic

hormone, a further use for it was found to fatten up livestock and chickens and is **still** used today for this purpose. That is why it is not safe to eat non-organic, hormone-treated meat in the United States. Twenty-one nations currently have a ban on the use of this chemical in food and fifteen countries refuse to import American meat because of it. (Paavlo Airola, *Cancer the Total Approach*).

Interestingly, Tamoxifen, a drug prescribed to women to attempt to prevent Breast Cancer and to prevent recurrence in Breast Cancer patients, is a synthetic hormone derived from DES. Side effects of this drug are Endometrial Cancer, Uterine Cancer, Liver Cancer, and blood clots to the lungs that can be fatal. Some studies have shown damage to the eyesight as well. The National Toxicology Program found both conjugated estrogens (Premarin) and Tamoxifen to be known human carcinogens in a report they compiled in 2000. They found these hormonal chemicals caused Endometrial Cancer as well as other Cancers.

10. **Chemicals, and additives in the food supply***:* Sales of chemicals in the U.S. take precedent over health. The FDA allows twenty-eight hundred chemicals to be used on food in their ingredients, and ten thousand more in their processing. Many of these are known to be carcinogenic.

   During my first battle with a lump in my neck from the Acrylic paints I used in my studio, I found some chemists to discuss how my health had broken down. One fellow showed me a hard, transparent Acrylic sample about one-half - by two inches resembling a small piece of glass. To my horror, he put it in his mouth and proceeded to swallow it! "Why this product is perfectly safe," he said. "They use it to spray apples and cucumbers." He went on to explain that they used to use beeswax to spray vegetables and fruits, but it got too expensive.

I was horrified! Go to any local supermarket and you will see very glossy apples and cucumbers, as well as other shiny vegetables and fruits. It is very important not to eat these plastic-coated vegetables and fruits. The plastic is hardened and cannot be scraped or rinsed off even with special wash-products. You might as well eat the plastic bags in which you put your produce! Even peeling is not good enough, as skins are semi-permeable, thus allowing plastic inside. It's important to buy only mat, non-shiny vegetables and fruits, preferably organic. Farmer's markets and specialty organic markets are safer, though you still have to examine closely what you buy. As in polyurethane-coated breast implants, the body attacks plastic as a foreign intruder, breaking it down to the chemical toluene, a very noxious, dangerous turpentine-like solvent that causes liver Cancer in mice. I would never use the caustic solvent in my Art Studio!

11. **Silicone-Gel Breast Implants and Saline Implants in Silicone Envelopes**; A horror story rivaling any subject Edgar Allan Poe would write about, breast implants for either cosmetic enhancement or breast reconstruction after mastectomy, have created severe health problems. Silicone-related symptoms commonly show up one year following breast implant according to *Doctor's Guide*, July 24, 2002. These complaints include Scleroderma, Autoimmune disease, joint pain, lumps of silicone throughout their body, chronic fatigue, capsular contraction (a hardening of scar tissue around the implant), and Breast Cancer. Many women have succumbed after years of debilitating symptoms and disease as their bodies desperately try to fight off these "foreign invaders."

    Implants, first introduced in the sixties, were known to leak before they were sent out into the marketplace. The subsequent lawsuits that have inundated Dow Chemical and other manufacturers of these implants, in the nineties, from sick and dying women, have not eliminated the demand for this dangerous procedure.

    Silicone Gel is an industrial material commonly used in the manufacture of electronic circuit boards. With a catalyst added, it is marketed as a window and door sealant and ceramic tile caulking. Recently when my bathroom full-length mirror fell off the door and crashed onto the floor, the workman who replaced it used silicone as a strong-smelling glue to attach the new mirror!

Artists have used the gel as a paint medium. I bought some to try, but after reading the label, I decided the gel was too dangerous for studio use. (Contains ammonia and if gotten in the eyes, call for immediate medical attention.)

Saline-breast implants are no safer as they come in silicone envelopes. The actress Sally Kirkland gives lectures warning of the dangers of saline, which gets moldy after some months within the body, leaking the contaminated water and mold throughout the system. Her implants also moved around, one sliding downward, turning her appearance into that of a freak, while robbing her, simultaneously, of her precious health.

12. **Preservatives in food, BHT, Nitrates:** It's important to read food labels. Brand-name breakfast cereals, popular with children, commonly use BHT as a preservative. This is Butylated Hydroxytoluene. Here again we meet up with Toluene, the toxic, turpentine-like thinner used in plastics that I consider too dangerous for my art studio use. It can lead to possible adverse effects of elevated cholesterol levels, allergic reactions, liver damage, infertility, sterility, behavior problems, loss of Vitamin D, a weakened immune

system and increased susceptibility to Cancer-causing substances. Toluene is also a substance found in the body after the above-mentioned breast-implant insertion. It is very important for one's health to avoid any products containing BHT!

Nitrates are found in processed meats, sausage, and hot dogs. This chemical has been proven to evolve within the body into nitrosamines, which are extremely carcinogenic, and can cause Cancer anywhere within the body. Children eating a steady diet of hot dogs have been found to have a high rate of leukemia, Cancer of the white blood cells.

13. **Smog and environmental carcinogens**: Exposure to air pollution in U.S. cities accounts for sixty thousand deaths annually according to a study at the Harvard School of Health. Many of the chemicals such as gasoline additives, exhaust fumes, and industrial pollutants can be found in the air as well as chlorine and fluoride in the water. Fluoride is a waste product of the aluminum and fertilizer industries. It was "sold" to Americans as a deterrent to tooth decay when, in actuality, it weakens our teeth and bones. It is legally put into our drinking water! These chemicals can damage cells, damage the DNA, as well as introducing toxins into the blood. Damaged cells that cannot be repaired by the body's defense mechanisms often turn Cancerous.

14. **Radiation**: Studies show that even low-dose radiation can cause Cancer over a long period of time. Even diagnostic X-rays used routinely by doctors and dentists have been implicated. Women exposed to radiation when Hiroshima was bombed often developed Breast Cancer. Cancer patients given radiation treatments often develop another Cancer twelve or more years later from these treatments, a case of today's cure being tomorrow's disease.

Radiation is high-velocity atomic particles that destroy any part of the body at which they are aimed. Genetic mutations and cell aberration can result from any exposure. Cumulative damage can occur throughout the body from multiple exposures throughout the years. Annual chest X-rays were finally discontinued when it was discovered they led to Thyroid Cancer.[3]

Annual mammograms as recommended for women age forty onward are not a great idea. Scientists knew when they sent out the machines that for every one-two Cancers they would detect, they would *cause* three- to-five others. Mammograms have a high rate of misdiagnosis, leading to missed Cancers in false-negatives and unnecessary biopsies in false-positives. Alternate diagnostic tools for Breast Cancer includes Thermography, MRI, and the AMAS blood test that can be gotten by submitting a blood sample to Oncolabs (1-800 9 CA-TEST). The blood test

---

3 Mendelssohn, Robert S. *Confessions of a Medical Heretic*, p.5.

is ninety-five percent effective at finding Cancer anywhere in the body.

A small vial of radioactive Cesium, a powerful source of gamma radiation used to treat Cancer and in food preserving, was lost somewhere in Northern California in 1993. The *Los Angeles Times* (Feb. 24, 1993) warned that clutching the container would produce skin burns within twenty-to twenty-five minutes, loss of hair within three or four days, and result in death after remaining in contact with the container in a week-to-ten days.

The dangers of X-rays can be found described in John Goffman's book on Breast Cancer prevention. He was a brilliant scientist in Berkeley who noted the dangers of radiation when he observed women in factories using the tip of their tongue to point brushes to paint radium dials in watches. These women slowly succumbed to Head, Mouth, Tongue and Throat Cancers.

I spoke with John Goffman on Breast Cancer at UC Berkeley on a panel on Breast Cancer prevention. He related how he lost his "golden boy" position in academia when he saw the serious dangers of radiation's use in the medical profession and began speaking up against it.

In 2002, a Danish meta-study of mammography failed to show that the X-rays provided any survival advantage in Breast Cancer.

15. **Cell Phones:** Evidence is piling up against putting a cell phone next to your ear. Electromagnetic radiation can heat cells damaging them. This may result in a small tumor called acoustic neuroma inside the ear. Cell phones may damage hearing ability. Also they may contribute to brain tumors if used excessively over a period of years.

16. *Physical, chemical, or mechanical injury or irritation:* Irritation or damage to the tissues over a period of time or physical trauma can cause Cancer. In an English study, Women age fifty to sixty-five with Breast Cancer in North Lancashire were found to have a link with physical trauma to the breast.[4]

    My sheep dog, Sandy, had a bad habit of chasing cars. He would repeatedly hit one side of his mouth. At age eleven, he developed Cancer on his jaw at just this spot. This affected his ability to eat and led to his death despite several operations to remove the Cancer.

    A nurse in rushing to answer the phone slammed her breast against a desk. She developed Breast Cancer in that spot some time after that. During that period, she was also going through a lot of emotional stress.

    A friend of mine also developed Breast Cancer in the spot where she was bitten by a tic.

    A pair of twins were studied by scientists, because one developed Breast Cancer, while one

4 "European Journal of Cancer Prevention", Aug. 1, 2002

did not. However, the one that did had a physically abusive husband who beat her in the chest area.

Physical trauma can often be healed over time by an effective and vigorous immune system. That system can be slowed or broken down by emotional problems and depression leading to a higher probability of Cancer.

Chemical damage from Chemotherapy drugs can lead to both heart problems and more Cancer down the line. Secondary Cancers and leukemia can result from this form of "treatment."

17. *High animal protein diet:* It is a dangerous myth that we need a lot of meat and dairy products. Over-eating meat and dairy fats are known causes of Cancer. A panel of the American Institute of Cancer Research convened in 1997, found animal fats in the diet to increase Cancer risk. An Indian Medical Journal, four thousand years old, lists Cancer. The cause is ascribed to "overeating dairy foods." Animal fats will accumulate and clog not only the arteries leading to cardiovascular disease, but the cells as well, leading to Cancer. It is a dangerous myth that we need a lot of meat to build strength. Meat and dairy fats are known to increase the risk of tumor development.

18. *Unusually severe stress:* People with lowered ability to deal with the stresses of everyday life, those with worries and fears and severe emotional

conflicts, are more susceptible to Cancer. The immune system actually shrinks in physical size under long-term chronic stress, even if the stress is imagined. The body then is then more vulnerable to unchecked growth of mutated cells.

19. *Emotional loss:* High on the list of stress inducers are the death of a spouse, divorce, and separation. I witnessed this phenomenon myself when a neighbor, who at age sixty-two was a jocular, robust, healthy man, deeply devoted to his older wife, became anxious when his wife fell ill. He did heavy yard work daily, digging and planting. When she died, he changed radically before my eyes. "Did you know my wife died?" he would ask me everyday as I walked past. Dispirited and confused, he seemed to waste away quickly, and within two months this very healthy man was dead of heart failure. Emotional loss and emotional turmoil is the number one stress and I believe an important causation of Cancer.

20. *Feelings of helplessness or hopelessness:* Loss of hope for a rewarding life and lack of enthusiasm for living, for getting up in the morning, creates depression. During a depressed state, the immune system actually shrinks in size and begins to shut down. We need to take positive steps toward solving difficult situations, however small those steps might be. Every attempt, even if it fails, will empower you and subsequently empower your immune system.

21. *Unhappy childhood leading to problematic adulthood:* According to O. Carl Simonton, the father of visualization, Cancer often strikes those who feel rejected by one or both parents during childhood. Psychologist Dr. Laurence Le Shan, noted that his Cancer patients often reflected a deep, basic feeling of rejection that had seemingly always been with them. Because of a current setback, we may fall into despair. The resulting depression and dejection stops or slows the immune system that cannot offer us protection from the bizarre cells that cause tumor growth.

22. *Some viruses:* Although we can't "catch" Cancer, one form of virus, the Rous Sarcoma, was shown to cause Cancer in chickens as early as 1910.

23. *Depression:* Loss of reasons to get up from your bed and start the day, to be able to create a meaningful life for yourself, to "sing your song," becomes the psychological undermining of the body paving the way for Cancer according to LeShan. He quotes Auden in calling Cancer, "foiled creative fire." In my case it was a combination of financial stress from the recession when my art stop selling and an emotionally disturbing relationship that, I believe, led me to be vulnerable to Cancer. I also was careless about my diet, overeating meat to try to compensate for my emotional loss.

When we review these causes: high-fat animal protein diet, overweight, miracle hormone drugs for menopause and birth control, hormones and pesticides in foods, air pollution, toxic chemical exposure, breast implants, emotional loss causing depression, and chronic stress, it is no wonder that one out of three women and one of two men will contract Cancer during our lifetime. While there is practically no way of avoiding at least some of these stresses, there are ways of protecting ourselves before acute damage to our cells results in disease. There is also a way we can heal the damage naturally. This is what this book is about. We will only make progress in our quest to conquer Cancer when we change our attitude toward it, take responsibility for the decline and deterioration of our health, and do the essential work necessary to rebuild it.

Let's look at the positive side before we close this chapter—some factors that can help us to avoid Cancer and rebuild our health:

1. A low-fat mostly vegetarian diet (fish is a good Cancer-fighting protein).

2. Weight control—reaching and maintaining our ideal weight.

3. Positive attitude. Being happy. Enjoying our work.

4. Having children before age thirty and breast-feeding them.

5. Having a religious or spiritual practice.

6. Once a month fasting or under-eating for a day.

7. Learning how to handle stress so as not to take it out on the body.

8. Group therapy when we have problems.

9. Good marriage.

10. Expressing our feelings (especially not holding onto anger and resentment).

11. Limiting our exposure to X-rays, chemicals, and smog.

12. Regular vigorous exercise, preferably one hour a day, five or six days a week.

13. Regular self-breast exams, self-examination of ones body looking for abnormalities, such as moles that get bigger, skin abnormalities, lumps in the lymph nodes, tumors, changes in bowel habits, unexplained pains or fatigue.

14. Turning down technological "miracles" that haven't had a twenty-year follow-up study or have negative studies such as birth control pills, estrogen replacement therapy, HRT, breast implants, and routine X-rays including mammography. All are potentially carcinogenic.

15. Protecting ourselves from mechanical or physical injury.

16. Learning how to self-heal our bodies, including how to rid one's body of tumors using natural means.

In summary, taking responsibility for one's own health, instead of waiting for the magic "cure" that never seems to be in sight, will be what finally makes inroads into the alarming Cancer mortality statistics. KNOWLEDGE IS POWER. When we finally wake up and realize that Cancer doesn't hit us "out of the blue," but is the cumulative result of our depressed mental and emotional state, along with our everyday habits as to how we treat or mistreat our bodies, we will make progress against this most feared disease. You can start today to prevent, heal, or prevent recurrence of Cancer. "They" can't do it. But **you** can. Depend on yourself to reinforce your will to live, strengthen your immune system, and to ride onto the road to health and stay on it. Life is our most precious gift.

CHAPTER 3

Defying the Prognosis

EVERY YEAR DURING Labor Day, Lorraine Rosenthal's Cancer Control Convention is held in Los Angeles. Each year, a line of people form to tell their story as to how they defied their doctor's prognosis and overcame their Cancer using all, or mostly all, natural means. These people are proud and happy; many have been Cancer-free for many years despite the doctor's gloomy prognosis. The year 2002 the Cancer Convention was particularly heartwarming when a little girl dressed in a lacy white dress, babbling happily away, took the stage with her parents.

YOUNG TORI'S SURVIVAL

Tori Moreno presented a miracle of survival. A breech baby who kept rotating around and around in Kim, her Mother's womb, she finally was born by Caesarian section. No one noticed anything wrong with her at birth. "She looked perfect," gushed her father, Roman. Her scores on reflexes, coloration and body proportion were all 9.9 out of ten. The only hint that anything was wrong after she came home from the hospital was that Tori's left eye would stay open when she cried, earning her the nickname of "one-eyed Jack." It was a joke until she was five or six weeks old when she seemed to have trouble tracking things with her eyes.

There seemed to be something wrong with the left side of her face. So her parents took her to the pediatrician. Dr. Albert Lee didn't think anything serious was wrong, but set up an appointment with a neurologist, who at first didn't suspect anything and asked Kim if she was a first time Mom. Finally he noticed something and ordered an MRI scan. Still, he didn't think it was anything to worry about.

Tori went from the MRI to the intensive care unit on a gurney. The nurses were whispering. The suspense was unbearable. Finally the doctor told them that Tori had a tumor in her brain stem. A surgical team was being assembled. She would be transferred to an emergency hospital and have surgery in the morning. He made it clear that anything involving brain surgery in an infant is extremely serious and dangerous. He said she needed surgery or she would die. She had a very rare and life-threatening tumor, "the worst glioma they had ever seen," aggressive and fast growing. There is no cure for this tumor in conventional medicine. The best doctors could hope for is to remove all or most of the tumor and wait for its almost inevitable re-growth within weeks or months.

The tumor turned out to be deep inside the brain stem and inoperable. "I'm sorry there's nothing I can do for you," the neurosurgeon apologized. The tumor had traveled throughout her brain stem, becoming intertwined with normal tissue. An oncologist told the parents that she might die at any time. The Oncologists told them that rarely did they come across a case in which they felt they could do nothing.

That's when the parents decided to look around for Alternatives. They searched the Internet and went to bookstores and finally found Dr. Stanislaw Burzynski, an Alternative doctor in Houston, Texas. Their insurance company refused to pay for the treatment he offers at his clinic. In fact, Dr. Burzynski, who was present at the Cancer Convention, a bright-eyed, vigorous looking man, has been harassed and persecuted by the FDA for his unconventional treatments, even though they often work! He is an upbeat man, not one who looks at all like a person who has been criminally indicted for healing terminally ill patients Alternatively. He uses Antineoplastons, a now synthesized substance that originally was derived from human urine. Peptides found in urine, can apparently help a Cancer patient heal. After a week, Tori's parents saw much improvement. Her eyes began tracking things normally, she sucked properly on her bottle, her eyes lost some of the droopy look and her left eye started blinking.

The Oncologists were astounded, as they had never seen a patient who had no chemotherapy or radiation survive more than a few weeks with a tumor like Tori's. When Tori became a bouncing baby, just over one year old, her Oncologist admitted that she was doing great! Her tumor had reduced by *seventy percent.*

Dr. Burzynski postulates that there is a secondary biochemical defense system that kicks in after the immune system fails to catch and conquer Cancer cells and a tumor forms. To get this second-layer defense system to "kick in," he uses a natural substance, human urine, an old folk remedy. Martha M. Christy used this to heal herself of Cancer and then wrote a book, *Your Own Perfect Medicine: The Incredible Proven Natural Miracle Cure that Medical Science Has Never Revealed.*

Dr Burzynski now synthesizes amino acids found in urine in his laboratory to give his Cancer Patients astounding results. His incurable patients, given up by the medical establishment, get well.

Norman Cousins, a distinguished writer who healed himself of an incurable disease with laughter, wrote of attempting to look up "Healing System" in the UCLA Biomedical Library. He could find nothing listed. Perhaps he was looking for this biochemical defense system that medical literature ignores.

I admire Dr. Burzynski who has fought it out with the FDA and has been in and out of court for years. He has helped thousands of people with Cancer recover their health. His story can be found in the book, *The Burzynsi Breakthrough: The Most Promising Cancer Treatment and the Government's Campaign to Squelch It*, by Thomas D. Elias (Lexikos, Nevada City, California, 2001).

THE HEALING SYSTEMS

I also concur with his findings of a secondary healing system that has to "kick in." In my own experience it involves the cells called cytokines that buzzed around like bees in my breast attacking the tumor. Meanwhile, the cells called pyrogens, or heat cells, heated up my breast until it turned red and hot, using the time-honored tool, fever, to obliterate Cancer. Inflammation of both my left breast and my left arm occurred, the lymph fluid swelling my left arm to the point of temporary paralysis, turning it into cement while the lymph fluid cleaned out my breast and heat-shock proteins protected my other cells during this spectacular reaction. Only my left breast, the one with the tumor and my left arm were affected. Although it was terrifying, this reaction was temporary, lasting only one day. I did my routine, swimming of one mile through it, using one arm to propel myself through the water.

Had I gone to a breast surgeon during that crucial time of my healing, he or she would have pronounced the disease Inflammatory Breast Cancer, believed to be a rare and dangerous form of the disease and given me a prognosis of two to eighteen months to live! Also I would have been given a "ninety-eight percent terminal" prognosis statistic.

Because fever is one of the least understood healing reactions, it is viewed with horror and fear. Fever is considered bad and drugs are given to combat it. Inflammation is also considered treacherous, and anti-inflammatory drugs abound. Yet Hippocrates, the Father of Medicine, acknowledged fever as a tool the body uses to heal disease. While it is frightening to observe any fever or inflammation, we must recognize the body's tools and support them by going through this temporary situation. It takes courage, stamina, and hope to get through any disease. Cancer takes a Herculean strength. You have to be very determined to get through it. *You have to really want to get well.*

Carrot juice was preferable to me over urine. Carrot juice plus my health program, MOTEP, worked equally well as urine-derived Antineoplastons. The smell and taste is also much better!

DR. MATTHIAS RATH'S ALTERNATIVES

Dr. Matthias Rath also has a special program for Cancer, the most feared disease. He once worked with the eminent scientist, Dr. Linus Pauling. He uses Vitamin C, and the amino acids L-lysine and L-proline for his Cancer patients. These are natural amino acids that are the building blocks of collagen and elastin fibers. L-lysine prevents digestion of collagen by blocking sites where enzymes attach, making this nutrient critical in preventing the degradation of connective tissue. Vitamin C and L-lysine, although they are essential for life, are not produced by the body. He also has his patients drink green tea, which contains Epigallocatechin Gallate or EGCG. The other supplements he recommends are Selenium, an anti-oxidant that is important in the defense system and suppresses tumor promotion and early stages of tumor progression through the inhibition of angiogenic enzymes, and N-acetyl-cysteine, a powerful antioxidant that is essential in the production of glutathion. Arginine, an essential amino acid and Copper and Manganese are also recommended supplements. At his presentation in downtown Los Angeles, he had a Lung Cancer patient speak who had healed from simply taking the above listed supplements.

Clearly the route of the future is healing Cancer utilizing natural substances instead of damaging and mutilating the body with "aggressive" surgery, chemotherapy, and radiation. "Cutting–edge" technology has been a complete and dismal failure in lowering Cancer mortality.

A natural approach to healing Cancer has been steadily gaining ground during the thirty years Lorraine Rosenthal has persevered with her Alternative Cancer Control Convention. In the following pages you will meet various people who approached Cancer using unconventional, natural means and not only got well, but improved their life. They continue to live a healthy life without "recurrence." Many tried the "conventional" route first to no avail.

LOREN'S Prostate CANCER

One such individual who turned to Alternative therapies is Loren. A scientist who overcame his Prostate Cancer, Loren calls Cancer "a socially accepted form of suicide." The subconscious mind has issued a death wish, he believes. He is now fifty-eight years old and lives in a beautiful part of the desert called Joshua Tree. After the medical treatment for Prostate Cancer that he had in 1994, his remission lasted two years. At that time, he had a relapse that he describes as "most dangerous" because the tools the Medical System uses "don't work" on recurrences.

Loren is an inventor and investigates bioelectrical energy that the body produces to move the cells and regulate metabolism. He utilized a water purification machine that mimics metabolism and did "energetics" and detoxification to purge his body of wastes. He took vitamins and minerals. "Better get well," he told himself. He feels his work isn't done. He incorporated many herbs and supplements into his diet such as Saw Palmetto, Green Tea, Pectin from grapefruit, Beta Carotene, Quercitin, Vitamin C, Acidolpholous, Glutamine, and Co-Q-Ten. He found that men over fifty have more estrogen than their wives and used flax-seed oil and Curcumin found in the spice, Turmeric, to balance his Testosterone/Estrogen hormones. He feels the Medical thinking has it "Bass-Ackwards." The hormone therapy they recommend is estrogenic.

"That is the same for women," I observe. They give women with Breast Cancer who are over estrogenic, Tamoxifen that acts like estrogen! They don't test the hormones, which is simply accomplished, with a saliva test to see why they are out-of-balance. Tamoxifen is a derivative of DES, a dangerous estrogen that was given to women to prevent miscarriage and resulted in Ovarian and Cervical Cancers in their daughters. It was finally taken off the market. But now they are finding a new use for it. They want to use carcinogenic and estrogenic chemicals it to "cure" Cancer!"

Loren laughed. He feels that the only way to get well is to balance the hormones, first testing the balance with a saliva test. He used Melatonin to re-balance his hormones. The future is in Natural Prostate cures, he believes. He has been well ever since. I spoke to him in 2001.

DOLORES' OVARIAN CANCER

After a routine gynecological examination in June of 1999, Dolores, now sixty-six was found to have Ovarian Cancer. The doctor had done a routine palpation and found "something." Dolores subsequently had surgery and believed that the doctor "got it all."

However, after a year and a half, she experienced a recurrence. The doctors recommended chemotherapy and radiation. Her defiance of this "treatment" comes through in her strong "No" that punctuates a normally soft voice that has a decidedly youthful ring to it. "This is all the Doctor knows," she explains.

She found a "Natural Oncologist," in Solana Beach, Ca. who treats her with vaccines, Laetrile from the bitter almond, Vitamin D and other supplements. She went on a Vegan diet and eats mostly raw fruits and vegetables, cooked beans, and whole grains. She eliminated sugar, all dairy foods, white bread and meat and eats only sprouted bread. She also incorporated flaxseed oil and Pau D'Arco.

She walks miles every day and gives all the "glory to God."

"I am well because of my faith in Him," she explains.

LEAH'S BREAST CANCER

Another strong-minded survivor, Leah learned to take care of herself. She was diagnosed with Breast Cancer in August, 1995 with a biopsy. A friend told her about the Stella Maris Clinic in Tijuana. She was open to alternative suggestions because she had seen a friend experience a recurrence after three surgeries and months of Chemotherapy. When her doctor at Kaiser recommended a mastectomy, she said "no." Her voice reverberates with strength as she told me her niece would object to her alternative route to healing. "I made up my mind." Her niece insisted she get a second opinion, so she did go to UCLA where they concurred with the mastectomy recommendation given to her by her first doctor.

"I don't believe in surgery as a healing modality," Leah says firmly. "Tell people to try the Holistic approach first."

She was turning sixty-five and believed her ability to survive depended on her healing choices. She has been well since the diagnosis and her alternative route to healing twelve years ago.

She did a lot of reading in the alternative healing area. At the clinic they did lymph massage, coffee enemas, juicing and herbs. She went on a diet of mostly raw organic fruits, vegetables and juices, combined with cooked whole grains to detoxify her body. She learned to meditate. Her attitude adjustment was very important, she believes. "You must be positive," she emphasizes. Most of all she explains, "Lifestyle change is paramount!"

Leah's husband died of heart problems; she feels he was over-medicated. "I tried to talk him out of taking all those pills, but there is only so much you can do. You can explain, try to get them to read a few books. In the end he kept taking them and I believe it weakened his immune system."

She still has financial difficulties.

"How do you stay well with all the stress you have?" I asked her.

"I have a new attitude now. Stress is 'out there' and I'm in here," she said firmly. Then she added plaintively, "Please get the word out! We are so invested in the surgery, chemotherapy, radiation and the drug route, the hospitals, the "conventional treatment," that we don't see the truth. The Doctors can't make us overcome Cancer. *We have to do it ourselves.* Cancer is within us and we have the power within to get well!"

"Exactly," I agreed. I had found that out in my own self-healing eighteen years ago.

ANN'S BREAST CANCER

Another strong survivor, Ann is 56 and was diagnosed with Breast Cancer in the left breast in July 2001. She opted for surgery to remove a .5-centimeter tumor. They then prescribed chemotherapy and radiation. She was working with a world-renown Oncologist. He talked her into arranging for chemotherapy but made the date a month down the line to give her some time to think about it.

Ann is a Buddhist who practices chanting. She began chanting up to three hours every day trying to make her decision as to what to do. She knew four educated, intelligent people who lost their lives doing the medical treatment for Cancer.

Her friend Kay had Stage Four Breast Cancer, and after months of chemotherapy and radiation, the Cancer came back. She also developed "Chemo-brain," a partial destruction of her memory. "Her mind was in a fog," she said. Talking to her celebrated Oncologist, he agreed that you may lose ten percent of your I.Q from doing Chemotherapy besides the gastrointestinal damage, hair loss, mouth sores, and worst of all the heart damage that these toxic chemicals produce.

She began to avidly research her options. An intelligent woman who spent her life as a journalist writing for the *Seattle Times* and a Media Educator, Ann believed in forming her own opinions based on books, articles, journals, newspapers and the Internet as well as interviews. She started with books. Her readings began with *Dr. Susan Love's Breast Book*, continued to Susun Weed's *Breast Health*, and finally to Susan Moss's *Keep Your Breasts*! She calls it her "three Susan's reading program." She also viewed Dr. Lorraine

Day's, "Cancer Doesn't Scare Me Anymore," a video she ordered.

Finally she found a health magazine enabling her to make her final decision. An article in that journal stated that seventy-five percent of oncologists interviewed would not do Chemotherapy if they themselves were diagnosed with Cancer!

After weeks of research, she had made up her mind. She called her Oncologist and cancelled her Chemotherapy appointment.

The look of fright that comes upon her face as she relates this communicates what she is about to tell me. "I was scared, at first. Then I decided to take control of my life."

Ann has been married twice. Since then she has had other relationships. Her last relationship failed to end happily, a tragic turn of events that she feels contributed to her Cancer. "I was going to marry this fellow until I suddenly realized he didn't love me," she says sadly with a touch of anger. She is extremely careful about getting involved with men, as she lost a child through a divorce. She can't reunite with this baby, her daughter who is now grown, and tells me, "You can't imagine the heartbreak I feel. Both my husbands hate me," she says sadly.

"Cancer is tied to the emotions; it is an emotional disease," I explain. "Almost everyone I've talked to who has had Cancer had emotional problems, turmoil, and a huge emotional stress in their life before they got ill."

Ann agreed. She said the Cancer Personality Chapter in my book was most important to her. She feels that emotions are ignored in Cancer treatment in which they proceed as if you are a robot. "This message has to get out," she emphasizes. Ann especially urges people with Cancer to reach out and help others. She does this by Shakabuku, helping others to learn how to chant, reinvigorate their lives and receive "benefits." She also chants for others. Chanting is a form of prayer. Studies have shown that people have gotten well from Cancer merely by being prayed for by others.

When she refused Chemotherapy, Ann found her Oncologist to be condescending. However, she was firm and began the MOTEP program, substituting my immune-system building program for the Medical Protocol. After three months, she went back for a blood test. "It was perfect," she enthused. She was then told to go on Tamoxifen. Again she refused. She was told that she needed hormone therapy for her bones and did try Fosamex for three months but found it did not agree with her. Instead she found a natural calcium product and ate salmon as substitutes for Osteoporosis drugs.

She also found a Naturopath to work with. He concurred that the Medical Treatment for Cancer turns a healthy body into a weak and sickly one. It was his mission to help heal the body naturally. She has been well since, a slim and vibrant woman with exuberance and energy. And now she has an additional mission to help get the word out.

MYRNA OSWILL, FAMOUS CANCER SURVIVOR

Perhaps the most interviewed survivor of Cancer is Myrna Oswill, seventy-five, who I met at a Cancer fair in Thousand Oaks in a park-like setting. I was sitting at my booth when she stopped by.

"I'm in all the books," she told me frankly. A spry and

energetic woman who looks much younger than her seventy-five years, Myrna now practices alternative medicine with others. "I'm a healer," she announces proudly.

Back in 1972, thirty-six years ago, she was diagnosed with a biopsy as having Breast Cancer. She refused the recommendation: a mastectomy to remove her entire breast.

"Good luck," the surgeon said, dismissing her curtly.

She began investigating her alternative options. She found Dr Ernesto Contreas in Mexico and began Laetrile therapy. Laetrile is Vitamin B-17 highly concentrated in Apricot Pits but available in twelve hundred other foods, some of which are listed in the Appendix. Vitamin B-17, a natural form of chemotherapy that doesn't poison normal cells, is used by the T-cells, which aim the cyanide content of the seed or food into the Cancer cells. The Cancer cells then die, a process called apoptosis. The body is very intelligent and well equipped to fight Cancer if given the proper tools. Blasting the body with Chemotherapy drugs, derived from war chemicals used as a toxic weapon and banned by the Geneva Convention in 1929 because of the serious gastrointestinal damage and mouth sores they cause, does terrible damage to the body. Chemo kills all fast-growing cells including hair cells and stomach and intestine cells. It is extremely toxic. This explains the hair loss, gastrointestinal damage, vomiting and worst of all, heart damage and brain damage.

There is a natural alternative that works much better and is much safer. Vitamin B-17 causes no side effects except if over-eaten. Two-to-four apricot pits, available in health food stores, are all that is needed. Supplements of this vitamin were banned by the FDA because they did not want the competition for their "blockbuster" Chemotherapy drugs that represent billions of dollars a year.

Myrna also believes that the mind plays a major role in Cancer. She believes the spirit is also of the utmost importance in this degenerative disease.

"Did you have a lot of stress?" I asked her.

"Cancer people always do," she stated flatly. "I had distress with both my husband and my children."

"How did you get well?" I asked her.

"You have to change your life," she said bluntly. "I had to change and get out from under the stress I was experiencing. Then I also changed my diet and began to seriously exercise. I do a lot of gardening in the morning. I get up early to do it—six a.m. I do a lot of walking and with it deep breathing exercises." She demonstrates her healing breath techniques for me as I marvel at this spry woman who was anything but an "old lady."

"This is the secret to a long-life, " she concludes, "spiritual rituals, changing eating habits and doing active and oxygenating exercise."

Off she went to the other booths at a rapid pace while I watched in awe at this wonderful, now famous Cancer survivor of thirty years. I marveled at her strong will and her ability to take her healing into her own hands and take a natural route to healing her Breast Cancer. It must have been especially difficult thirty years ago when mastectomy was the standard treatment. Her Doctor's cold, rejecting attitude was probably "standard treatment" also.

A BEAUTY SURVIVES CANCER

I sat at my booth in the park in Thousand Oaks Cancer Fair with my books and awaited the next eye- opening, amazing story. Next came Margaret, a stunning brunette, looking as if she had never had a sick day in her entire life. She wore motorcycle-type clothes, a revealing black vest, tight black pants and leather boots, all wrapping around a stunning figure. She reminded me of a young Elizabeth Taylor in "Butterfield 8."

I was stunned to find out that she had survived three recurrences of Breast Cancer. First diagnosed in 1993 of Invasive Intraductal Breast Cancer, she was strongly recommended to receive a mastectomy followed by chemotherapy and radiation.

"Let's hold off," she said, much to the Oncologists consternation. "Let's find another approach."

She went on a raw food diet and did a liver cleanse program. After three months she opted for an excision of her lump. They found no Cancer.

But in 1995, she had a second primary tumor. She went to the top expert, Dr. Susan Love. Her nipple had by then become inverted, a treacherous sign. This scared her. She agreed to a lumpectomy followed by radiation and chemotherapy for six months. This, she thought, would finally solve the problem.

It didn't work for long. In 1999, she was diagnosed with a recurrence. This time she refused all medical treatment. "Enough is enough," she decided. Though she consented to another Lumpectomy, she refused all other forms of standard medical treatment. She did a more intense program of natural healing including Acupuncture, Tibetan Herbs, and white-blood cell support through exercise, visualization and spiritual exercises such as chanting and prayer.

"I'm fine. I feel wonderful," she says. "My tests are clean. I have no Cancer."

She frowns. "The doctors won't speak to me. They want to give me more drugs and radiation. My clean tests perplex them. It's not what they learn in Medical school."

Margaret was visibly upset. "It's about the money that goes in the Pharmaceutical Pockets, not about getting well. If you want to get well there are ways. But you have to do it yourself."

TAKING A NON-CONVENTIONAL PATH

I was in awe of this stunning, courageous woman. Cancer patients that not only defy the disease, as she did three times, but defy the Conventional Medical Treatment are brave beyond imagination. The character traits I have found in interviewing these survivors include an amazing strength, a strong belief in their own healing abilities, a willingness to stake their life on those beliefs, and a strong drive to help others. They truly are an inspiration as well as pioneering the way toward a new paradigm of Cancer healing.

At the Cancer Control Convention in 2002, I also met Kari. At age forty, she had been recently diagnosed with Breast Cancer with a biopsy, and was an intelligent and curious seeker of alternative information. She bought my book and expressed willingness to go on the MOTEP healing program.

She would be my next "Clinical Trial." Her story will continue throughout this book.

I always leave Alternative Cancer conventions and fairs in a state of awe while thinking back on the many inspirational stories of the very strong and inspirational survivors I meet. They beat the odds and they did it their own way. You can too!

CHAPTER 4

The MOTEP Program—
Travelling the Road Back to Health

THE ROAD BACK TO health is taken as soon as you take the first step. That step is taking responsibility for your health.

This does not involve any blame, guilt, or misgivings. But it does involve the willingness to change any and every part of your life that may have contributed to your Cancer. Sometimes it does take a major trauma or crisis to get us to face our negative, self-destructive habits. We may have easily fallen into a rut, using harmful habits to escape the reality of our lives.

I found that although it took tremendous self-discipline to get myself into this program, the efforts I made to restore my health began paying off very quickly. My two tumors that had probably taken at least a year or two to grow were gone in only two months. I had to stay on my program another seven months before I had rebuilt my body into the glowing, vibrant health I still feel today, eighteen years later.

I grew to love this program so much that I am still on it. The rewards are great not only in my health and personal appearance, but also the tremendous successes I have achieved since I stared down death. The Buddhists like to turn obstacles into a springboard for opportunities for growth. If you look at Cancer as a "cure" for neurotic, self-destructive behavior then Cancer can actually be a benefit. If you look for a reason to do what you always wanted to do for yourself, for permission to ask for what you want and need, to be able to tell people how you feel, then Cancer can, indeed be your "turning point."

THE MOTEP HEALING PROGRAM

Without further fanfare, here is MOTEP—Marathon Olympic Tumor Eradication and Prevention program:

1. A low-fat mostly vegetarian diet. I included fish.

2. Under-eating slightly for a period of a month. Lots of nutrients can be consumed by juicing, eating vegetables, fruits, whole grains, nuts and seeds, and vitamins, while at the same time cutting calories.

3. Weight control—reaching and maintaining our ideal weight.

4. Elimination of all pharmaceutical pills and drugs that aren't life essential.

5. Increase in Vitamin supplements (A, Selenium, B, C, E, Calcium, Zinc and foods containing Laetrile (see appendix).

6. Fresh juiced carrots (about eight) and fresh juiced oranges (about four) every day.

7. Eight hours sleep per night and a half-hour nap during the day.

8. Regular, vigorous exercise, preferably one hour a day, five or six days a week.

9. Positive attitude. Being happy. Enjoying our work. Building positive, loving relationships.

10. Having a religious or spiritual practice. Visualization, chanting, prayer, (morning and evening).

11. Breast-feeding our children, preferably having them before age thirty.

12. Once a month juice fasting, or under-eating for a day.

13. Learning how to keep stress "out there" without taking it out on our body.

14. Group therapy when we have problems or after a major emotional loss.

15. Good marriage or relationship.

16. Expressing our feelings (especially not holding onto anger and resentment).

17. Limiting our exposure to X-rays, chemicals, and smog.

18. Making it a point to help and encourage others.

19. Giving love to others, and to yourself, generously.

20. Smiling and laughing as much as possible (inspired by Norman Cousins).

Those are the "top twenty" steps of my MOTEP program. In addition I have added a few others for this new book on healing all Cancers.

21. Regular self-breast exam, skin exam, and a relationship with a doctor who can diagnose Cancer without invasive procedures.

22. Turning down technological "miracles" that have proven carcinogenic, such as birth control pills, estrogen replacement therapy, HRT, breast implants, routine yearly mammograms and unneeded CAT scans that involve regular radiation exposure. The breasts are exquisitely sensitive to radiation. Physicists are now warning against CAT scans for healthy people because it delivers hundreds of times the radiation of a chest X-ray. (*L.A. Times*, September 16, 2002). Mammograms have not slowed the Breast Cancer epidemic nor lowered the mortality rate. Protecting our bodies as much as possible from mechanical or physical injury.

23. Inducing in yourself a feeling of well being no matter what your actual circumstances are.

24. Asking for help and support from others instead of playing loner.

25. Learning how to self-heal our bodies, including how to rid the body of tumors by natural means.

26. Having absolute faith in MOTEP and your body's own abilities to heal any disease.

27. A strong determination to survive, will to live, and a longing to share your experience with others.

BELINDA TRIES THE MOTEP PROGRAM

"It works!" The jubilant voice on other end of the telephone line was Belinda, age thirty-seven. She is a dynamic young woman who was referred to me by Pamela Kelly who gave me the opportunity to speak to her UCLA women's study classes when my first book on Breast Cancer was still only a spiral-bound manuscript.

Belinda is a high-risk candidate for Breast Cancer. Her aunt had died of the disease at age forty-seven. Her mother had also fought the disease but successfully. Belinda had gone to the Doctor for her annual check-up. The mammogram showed a thickening of the breast, a probable sign of Cancer. She was told to come back for a biopsy within thirty days. We had to work fast!

I went over to visit Belinda, my first "clinical trial" volunteer. Granted, I did not have a clinic. But I believe the world's best clinic resides within our own body. We have a pharmacopoeia of drugs, hormones, tumor-suppressor genes, neuro-receptors, neuro-receivers, cytokines, pyrogens, leukocytes, T-cells, B-cells, natural killer cells, macrophages, phagocytes, and other white-blood cells as well as Tumor-necrosis factor, Interleukin, and Interferon— blood factors that can fight Cancer cells and even eliminate tumors. All we have to do is empower them and make the effort to help these Cancer fighters get into shape and into action.

Belinda was a dynamic, energetic woman who looked to me to be in quite a lot of turmoil and very distressed. Her appearance was a bit chaotic, her hair sticking out at ends and her outfit thrown together. I gave her a copy of the manuscript,(the first book was not as yet published), as I am not a doctor and can't give anyone medical advice. I did not comment on her distraught appearance. However, I did ask her some questions about her relationships. She said she had bad ones, problems with her Mother, her boyfriend, her boss—just about everyone in her life.

"It's important to your health to start healing these relationships," I told her. I also recommended lots of bright colored fruits and vegetables, orange, yellow, and dark green, that would be loaded with beta-carotene, plus lots of aerobic exercise, and began to teach her visualization techniques.

She was about to embark on a ten-day vacation in Mexico. This, I thought, would be the perfect "clinic" for her. And it was. She followed the MOTEP program enthusiastically. She exercised vigorously all day, doing swimming, scuba diving, sailing and running and walking on the beach. Away from her everyday stresses at work and her problem relationships, Belinda began to relax and find joy and an inner peace and the contentment she craved. She concentrated on eating beta-carotene and Vitamin C rich cantaloupe, mangoes, carrots, oranges, and dark green leafy vegetables. She eliminated most meat and dairy products, eating fresh fish instead. "I did visualization constantly, even when I was riding on the bus," she told me enthusiastically. "I visualized sharks eating any Cancer cells I might have. I visualized my breast growing healthy and shrinking back to normal."

Ten days later, she returned to Los Angeles. Her mother called in an anxious state, urging her to go back to the doctor and get her biopsy, though she wasn't due for twenty more days. Truly, my "clinic" was being turned into a fast-heal drive-through! It takes time to get well! But what can I do? I am only an author.

The doctor scheduled the appointment. A preliminary mammogram was again taken.

But much to the doctor's shock and amazement, the films were perfectly clear! "We wouldn't know where to cut," they told her. "Come back in four months."

Belinda was thrilled. In *only ten days,* she had cleared up the problems that had showed up in her Mammogram. She attempted to tell her doctor about my health program. However, the doctor refused to listen and brushed off this miraculous occurrence, this victory of my "clinical trial" as some sort of fluke! Truly, we have a way to go before the entire medical community can accept my program with an open mind. However, when the program became a book, some of the Medical community became surprisingly supportive. MOTEP had worked for Belinda extremely well and in only that amazingly short time! This is truly an achievement we were both very proud of. This amazing success has opened possibilities for all women with problem mammograms.

ANOTHER EARLY SUCCESS

My next "clinical" patient took the time and *was* patient. She healed her problem mammogram in four months, turning it to clear. In the future, perhaps, wise women will use the MOTEP program to try to reverse problem mammograms and heal their bodies for two to four months before they agree to any invasive tests such as biopsies or more even more drastic surgeries.

Most Alternative Practitioners are against biopsies because they create scar tissue that can actually up the risk of further Cancers. Invasive surgeries to explore the extent of the disease are also unnecessary and involve the risk of anesthesia, cutting into the body, infections, scar tissue, and drug side effects. Any surgery is extremely traumatic to the body and will necessitate the power of white blood cells to heal the wounds inflicted by the surgeon's knives. These white-blood cells that are so desperately needed to heal the Cancer are way-laid.

Why submit to exploratory surgery at all? If Cancer has begun to take inroads, a healing journey must be started immediately. Many people die during surgery because it is extremely violent and traumatic to the human body. Exploratory surgery is for the surgeons! Once again we become prey to a Medical Establishment's fund-raising efforts and experiments. Billions of dollars are raised by ineffective and destructive methods of diagnosing and treating Cancer. If these methods only work for less than half the patients for five years, what are we doing?

Looking at the lifetime of a Cancer patient who undergoes current treatments, rather than the five-year model, eighty percent will die with or from their original Cancer, in the same place or metastasized to other parts of the body, called recurrence. Some will die from a new type of Cancer. Yet, those who heal naturally usually stay well. I believe this is for two main reasons.

First, the person who takes responsibility and does a slow natural healing, changing their lifestyle and altering destructive habits, replacing them with positive health-enhancing ones, strengthens his or her immune system. Once it learns to heal Cancer, the immune system has that knowledge. Dendritic cells, guardians of the body, are nature's way of inducing immune response. They circulate and capture foreign proteins and present them to T-cells, which learn to recognize them. The T-cells then eliminate the invaders. A child who has Chicken Pox and gets well will probably never get it again as an adult.

Second, people who get well naturally are usually reluctant to "go back" to their old, destructive lifestyle. Cancer has taught them that the risks outweigh the "benefits." They gain a new appreciation for life and a new understanding of how the delicate balance of health can be altered over time to create a life-threatening situation. They have learned about stress and unhealthy habits that broke down their health. They are eager to share their knowledge with others. They want to help spread the word. They have found that Cancer has been a strange sort of "gift" in that they were forced to really look at themselves, their lifestyles, their eating habits, their goals, and their relationships and navigate toward a more positive direction. They are reborn. They have a new mission in their life to help others and this they do with great zeal and pride. They have found joy and strength and renewal in their life.

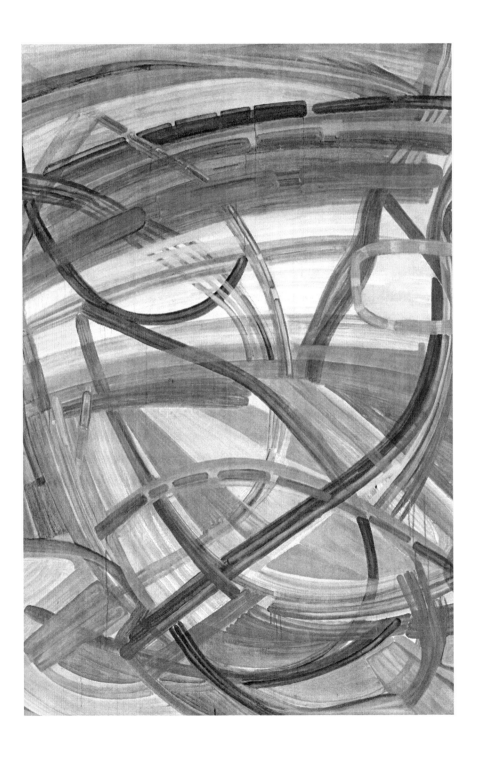

CHAPTER 5

You Are What You Believe

BEFORE WE GET into a deeper discussion of the MOTEP program, we need to look its most important element. That is the belief that what you are doing every day to steer your body back into the direction of health is going to eventually work.

This is the hardest part, of course, because it involves faith and trust in the body's resilience. As anyone who has survived Cancer can tell you, the body has amazing recuperative powers. The body has an incredible and varied arsenal of defense against Cancer. The T-Lymphocyte cells originate from the lymph glands and routinely destroy Cancer cells. They do this by squirting a bit of natural cyanide into the cells, a natural form of chemotherapy, from Vitamin B-17, the bitter taste in apricot pits and the other foods listed in the Appendix. The B-cells, from the bone marrow attack Cancer cells. Macrophages, like tiny "dust-buster" vacuums, swallow Cancer cells up. The most famous of these white blood cells is NK cells, or natural killer cells. These are the highly trained regiment cells called up for action.

If these cells fail, the next line of defense is blood factors. Tumor Necrosis Factor is what its name implies a blood factor that is designed to obliterate tumors. Interleukin, Interferon, and the newly discovered Angiostatin are also called into defense action.

If we really would try to understand tumors, we would see that they are desperately needed because they are trying to protect us! Tumors are not the enemy, nor are they the disease. They do not always need to be removed surgically. Cancer cells that begin to proliferate are caught in a cage of protective hard protein. Picture an egg with a hard shell protecting a chicken embryo, except this tumor shell is containing the Cancer cells. That is why Cancerous tumors are hard. Cancer cells are threatening the body, so a hard shell protective coating forms around them to wall them off. This protein coating cordoning off the Cancer cells also emits a hormone called Angiostatin, according to research done by Michael O'Reilly at Children's Hospital in Boston. This hormone courses through the bloodstream to wipe out micro-metastases. Only the tumor shell has the ability to make Angiostatin.[1]

Removing the tumor surgically often results in micro-scopic metastasis that ultimately overwhelms the patient. This happens for two reasons. First, the knife may cut into the tumor, breaking the shell and releasing the cordoned off Cancer cells, or spread them during the operation itself. Second, taking the tumor out, as in "lumpectomy" removes the body's ability to make Angiostatin to conquer the micro-metastases. Dr. George Crile, an early pioneer and advocate for limited Breast Cancer surgery noticed that removing the tumor often resulted in widespread Cancer. A nurse I spoke to who worked in Oncology for a decade, told me that when

---

1 Olson, James, S. "Bathsheba's Breast—Women, Cancer and History", Baltimore, John Hopkins University Press, 2002. P.253.

the surgeon operates on a tumor to remove it, the Cancer often spreads "like wildfire."

That is why I so strongly am in favor of what I call "Self-Lumpectomy." That is not using a knife, but de-toxifying and de-stressing the body to bring it back to a level of health that will enable these tumor-fighters to get back in the internal arena to fight and obliterate the tumor on their own. Bringing the body and mind back into full health will, according to my experience, result in the body discarding the tumor because it is no longer needed. You have brought the cells back to total health. You can even turn Cancerous cells back into normal cells!

So the first step is to believe in your own immune system and its miraculous powers to heal Cancer. You must empower them. This needs to be followed by a willingness to give your body what it needs to get well. This should be accompanied by a reluctance to place your health, completely and without questioning, into anyone else's hands. This includes handing your body over to an Oncologist, Surgeon, Doctor, or even a Healer, Chiropractor, or Guru without acknowledging that no one else can make you well. They can offer encouragement, and become a partner in your quest for health. But they can't make you well.

Only *you* can make the slow and gradual improvement from disease to full, vigorous health. These other people may or may not be able to help you, but basically it is up to you. Only you can heal your body. Only your own cells can do the job of turning your Cancer around back into full, joyful health.

KARI TURNS HER LIFE AROUND INTO HEALTH

Let's get back to Kari, age 40, whom I met at the Cancer Control Convention. She was diagnosed with Breast Cancer with a biopsy in her right breast where there was a tumor in the inner portion in August of 2002. She ultimately decided to utilize the MOTEP program to rid herself of a breast tumor without surgery, despite vociferous opposition from her relatives and friends. To bolster her belief system she uses affirmations she emphasizes are truly important. She realized that believing in her own healing powers was the key to getting well.

While exercising on the re-bounder, a small type of trampoline, she said aloud, "I am alive and well and totally free of Cancer." While walking her three miles a day and doing a variety of arm exercises simultaneously such as breaststroke and back crawl movements as if she were swimming, she affirmed, "I feel the tumor dissolving and disappearing. I am free and clear of all tumors."

Kari, after being diagnosed, was bombarded with advice from doctors, surgeons, her live-in boyfriend, relatives and well-meaning friends to go ahead with the Medical Treatment recommended — the surgery, chemotherapy, and radiation. She began by turning down the Sentinel Node Biopsy because it would involve injecting radioactive material into her body. She continued by going on the MOTEP program to see if she could bring her body back to health naturally.

Kari had damaged her body for years. Her childhood was spent in Norway where her environment was physically and emotionally cold. She describes her parents as non-emotional and stoic. She has two older brothers she does not feel close to. Both her parents were heavy smokers.

A beautiful tall woman with a shapely figure, she was rather lifeless and depressed, a colorless gray nondescript, fearful person when I met her. Since going on my program she has turned into a sparkling, lively and gorgeous lady with a mission — fighting for her life using natural means and a burning desire to help others when she achieves her goal.

Kari began smoking when she was eighteen finally quitting at age thirty-six. She also got into drugs—Marijuana, Speed, and Cocaine beginning at age eighteen and getting heavily into them by age twenty-three. She also began to drink and became an alcoholic in her thirties. Finally at age thirty-six she decided to go cold turkey, abruptly quitting drinking. Her life, she decided, wasn't working. She had had two abortions. She feels the abortions contributed to her Breast Cancer. Four years later she was diagnosed with the disease.

Her detoxifying program includes juicing. She bought a juicer in September after attending Lorraine Rosenthal's Cancer Control Convention, finding Dr. James Privitera and my book and meeting me. Her juices include a mixture of garlic, ginger, celery, carrots, parsley, and collard greens. She drinks two-and-a-half glasses daily. She also likes carrot juice spiked with ginger.

Her diet includes whole grains like barley and brown rice, vegetables and fruits and some fish and eliminates meat and dairy products. "I'm not going back to fast-food hamburgers!" she told me emphatically. After months on the program, she went to breakfast at a greasy spoon with her boyfriend. "I got totally sick," she later told me. "I just can't eat that way anymore!"

The momentous change, then, in Kari's life is a reticence to go back to her old, destructive lifestyle. Her energy was jump-started to begin to conquer her own Cancer along with a strong conviction that she can do it herself. "It's a recipe for health," she explains. "It makes sense."

So far, the progress she has shown besides the phenomenal change in her appearance to a healthy and vigorous woman extremely in shape is redness, burning and itching in her breast, a sign of healing mechanisms at work. She set a deadline for her healing for Thanksgiving. She was also willing to extend it to Christmas if need be. Kari's story will be continued in this book because I already feel she will be a victor. I usually can tell just by talking with these newly diagnosed people, if they have the core belief and inner strength to get well. Once you have this strength, in my own experience and others, it takes two-to-four months on the program to reverse a problem mammogram or dissolve tumors and see them completely disappear using entirely natural means. Belinda was a startlingly strong exception, returning to health in only ten days!

Kari began seeing Dr. James R. Privitera who did the blood-work on her. After two months on my MOTEP program and taking additional vitamin supplementation he gave her, he declared her past the critical stage and on her way to health. Her blood cells had changed from an abnormal shape to perfectly round. Her white blood cells changed from passive to very active. Dr. Privitera describes the blood of Cancer patients as "sticky." He can tell by the feel of the blood alone, if the person is heading down the hill toward Cancer! Seeing normal blood cells, he can tell that much of the work of healing has been accomplished. Kari *believed* she could turn her health around with her own hard work. This was the first step in her miraculous healing.

She still had the tumor in her breast, however, but he considered her way past the danger point. It will take at least two more months, I predicted, before her body will be ready for the "healing reaction" that will dissolve the tumor. More about Kari and a list of supplements she took will be in the next chapter.

BELIEVE IN YOUR HEALING POWERS

Stage four Cancers such as Orlan's take longer. Her Breast, Colon, and Lung Cancer took about eight months to stabilize. She is alive fourteen years later, working, traveling and on the lookout for a boyfriend, however, having originally been given a prognosis of three months providing she did extensive surgery. She did no surgery. Her belief in her body's ability to slowly regain her health never wavered.

Prayer, chanting, meditation and visualization are most important components of MOTEP. You are what you believe and what you want for yourself. Twenty minutes of prayer slows the heart rate, metabolic rate, and lowers the stress level of the person practicing spiritual activity. "If you believe you can heal, and you take responsibility, you can get well," Marius, an alternative healer who has worked with Cancer patients, says. Spiritual activities are of the utmost importance for anyone wanting to heal Cancer. Putting oneself in a spiritual place, in a trance as one chants, is an effective form of self-hypnosis. As you chant or pray or meditate, you can visualize your tumor shrinking and disappearing. You can visualize your own successes and can picture a happy life for yourself complete with abundance, with all of what you really want and need. You can produce a calm determination to enter a realm of perfect health. You can chant, pray, and send healing vibrations to others. In Buddhist practice, you also pray for your deceased relatives.

In the Universe, all our spirits are connected. You are not alone in your quest for health. Others will support you when they see you are determined to reclaim your health by your own efforts. Eventually the doctors will go along too. "I don't know what you are doing, but whatever it is keep it up," is the usual comment from physicians. A few don't want to know. But to my surprise, there are some very open-minded Doctors out there that are curious enough to start asking me questions. To my amazement, a retired surgeon sought out my studio, driving all the way from the Valley. He admitted he only got fifty-percent good results with surgery, losing the other fifty percent, and wanted to learn more about my healing program.

"The only thing to fear is fear itself," President Roosevelt said. While fear and intimidation are often used by the Medical Establishment to frighten a person diagnosed with Cancer into accepting destructive and mutilating treatment, doctors scaring patients by telling them the disease might spread (but it might also heal), fear can also be conquered by drawing on one's own self-will. We all have an inner strength we can access in time of major catastrophes.

VICTORS

The victorious people I have interviewed have strong convictions about getting well. They all can tell me point-blank why they got ill. There is no doubt in their mind that the (usually emotional) distress they went through and subsequent depression, the failure to give their bodies what they needed, and their own self-destructive habits created a weakened immune system allowing the Cancer to grow. Most of them tell me how their life wasn't working out, how they had emotional stress from deaths in the family, divorce, or tumultuous relationships, how self-destructive habits helped to create their diseased state.

Then their face lights up and their voice has a lilt as they tell me how they began juicing, taking herbs, eating semi-vegetarian diets with mostly organic foods, taking vitamin supplementation, began to exercise, incorporated spiritual activity, and came to the realization that their negative relationships needed to be mended or changed. They began to open up, going to therapy, joining a group and finally finding ways to help others. They found many new happy relationships and mended old ones. They learned how to express their anger, especially in self-defense. They came to grips with their grief over lost love ones and began a new direction in their lives. They changed vocations to something they truly loved and were avidly interested in. They took vacations to exotic places and spent time meditating and accessing their inner healing ability. They learned not to take mental stress out on their own physical body. They became generous with themselves and others, learning not to withhold. Their posture changed to being proud and upright. They gained new confidence and self-esteem. These triumphant individuals all have a new purpose in life—a profound interest in their own health and that of others.

Most of all they learned the greatest lesson of all: give the gift of love to yourself and to others. Love is the most healing emotion on the planet.

CHAPTER 6

Blood Story—A Portrait of Your Health

WHILE DOING A book signing in a small bookstore in Pasadena some years ago, I met Art who, after years of selling real estate with his parents, had gone back to school to study Alternative Medicine and Chinese herbs for healing. He introduced me to my blood story.

Taking a painless pinprick of my blood and looking under a dark-field microscope, he could see the image of my health. This is called Darkfield and Live Cell Analysis and is practiced by Dr. James R. Privitera. Dr. Privitera wrote the introduction to my Breast Cancer book and generously for this book too. Not only that, he was the only doctor who would do it without stipulating that I change parts of it. He says in his book, *Silent Clots—Life's Biggest Killers,* that, "The reality is that blood clots are the leading cause of death."

Not only that but the blood that shows clotting, shows Cancer. This surprising fact left me speechless—that a simple pinprick of the finger to obtain one drop of blood is all that is really needed. Rather than a dose of radiation from a Mammogram or Cat-Scan, or an invasive biopsy operation that might disfigure, infect, spread Cancer, and always creates scar tissue upping the chance of getting more Cancer, this was so easy, clear and inexpensive. Why isn't the medical community looking at blood?

WHAT YOUR BLOOD LOOKS LIKE DETERMINES YOUR HEALTH

Art gave me a chart showing various patterns of the blood and what they represent. On the next two pages you will see this graphic display. I found it fascinating. In Dr. Privitera's book, he shows more examples of patterns of red-blood cells called platelets and what diseases they represent. Art did my blood analysis at several different times.

At first, he found Rouleau, meaning a row of red corpuscles in French. The cells pile up in skewed skyscraper fashion like bent rows of coins, reminding me of the Slinky I played with as a child. This Rouleau pattern indicates poor oxygenation, causing fatigue, shortness of breath, bad digestion, edema, and low skin temperature. After working harder on my health for a month, I did another pinprick test with Art.

My blood looked normal! On the next two pages you can view the blood portraits that indicate various stages of health.

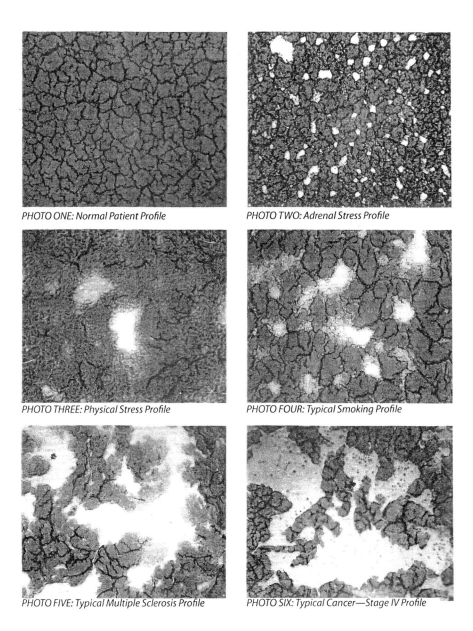

PHOTO ONE: Normal Patient Profile

PHOTO TWO: Adrenal Stress Profile

PHOTO THREE: Physical Stress Profile

PHOTO FOUR: Typical Smoking Profile

PHOTO FIVE: Typical Multiple Sclerosis Profile

PHOTO SIX: Typical Cancer—Stage IV Profile

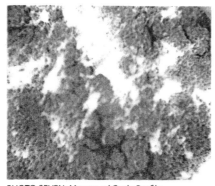

PHOTO SEVEN: Menstrual Cycle Profile

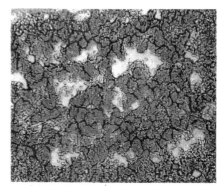

PHOTO EIGHT: Inflammation Profile

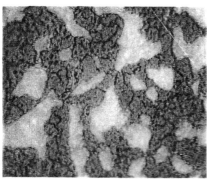

PHOTO NINE: Typical Severe Arthritic Profile

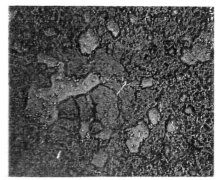

PHOTO TEN: Tuberculosis Profile

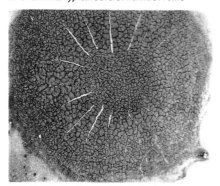

PHOTO ELEVEN: Hypercalcemia Profile

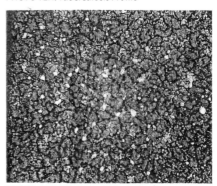

PHOTO TWELVE: Typical Allergy Profile

As you can see, Cancer has a specific blood profile that needs to be reversed back into normal. Also, you may note that removing the tumor does not change the blood profile. These portraits affirm that Cancer is always systemic illness. It is *never* a local disease involving only a tumor that can be cut out or Cancer cells that the surgeon can magically scoop out, convincing himself and the patient that he "got it all."

I think this is really of the utmost importance and why we have such a high rate of recurrence in Cancer-surgery patients. Even in Leukemia and Lymphomas where the white- blood cell count is way too high, it doesn't make sense, viewing these charts, to give Chemotherapy Drugs to wipe out the white blood cells. This may be a temporary quick fix, but when the blood goes back to its previous pattern, the Leukemia is said to have "recurred." The blood has not been supported by nutrition, exercise, and other health-enhancing practices, to bring it back to its normal pattern.

The second page of Blood Profiles shows different typical and atypical patterns of blood. Menstrual blood is unusual looking, inflammation is again involved in some bunching together of the red blood cells with some white-blood cells trying to aid the situation. In severe Arthritis, the red blood cells have almost become clumped ropes in a field of white blood cells. Tuberculosis looks grim and dark, Hypocalcaemia looks like very tightened and shrunken red blood cells and the Allergy profile shows a tweed pattern of white and red blood cells. These photos are a stunning confirmation of how our blood changes because of our own stresses, habits, internal toxins, and illnesses. Dr. Privitera and other Alternative Healers can see a portrait of your health simply by gazing at one drop of your blood under a microscope.

DR. PRIVITERA SEES KARI'S BLOOD CHANGE BACK TO NORMAL

Kari began going to Dr. Privitera in conjunction with doing the MOTEP program. "He's an M.D.," she explained. "That makes my relatives, boyfriend, and friends happier."

Because she was steadfastly doing the MOTEP program, taking scrupulous care of her body, Dr. Privitera saw faster results than he usually obtains. Kari changed her blood from a clotting pattern and inactive white blood cells to a normal pattern with active white blood cells, in less than two months! He was amazed that she reversed her severely abnormal blood pattern so quickly, but gave credit to the MOTEP program.

Dr. Privitera believes that one of the biggest causes of clotting is stress that causes nutritional deficiencies. In times of extreme stress, the adrenals put out Adrenaline and Corticosteroids that cause the blood to clot. Our bodies use up nutrients at a rapid rate causing nutritional deficiencies. Dr. Privitera determines what supplements are needed through looking at the blood through a dark-field microscope, analyzing the hair for mineral loss, and doing a Urine Indican test. He takes your underarm temperature to determine how well your thyroid is doing. He tells me that a diet of all raw food will often turn a thyroid problem around.

For Kari, he prescribed the following supplements: Borage Oil, Zinc, Iodine Drops, Thyroid, Vitamin C in Ester-C form, Mega Omega fish oils, CoQ-10, Immune Booster, Potassium Magnesium Citrate, Vascuzyme, Indoplex, Calcium D-Glucarate, Curcumin (available in Turmeric) and Cellfood (nascent oxygen and hydrogen).

In less than two months with the addition of supplements, Kari, using the MOTEP program had turned her blood back to normal. She still had the tumor, however. She still had work to do.

Dr. Privitera describes this situation as "stabilized Cancer" and notes that ridding the body of the tumor is *not* a requirement for a long life. He has had a patient who stabilized her Cancer without ridding herself of her tumor and lived on for *twenty-five* years finally dying in her eighties. Other patients such as Rose Alessio and Lena Lopez have stabilized their Cancers and live on despite the fact they still have evidence of Cancer!

KARI'S TUMOR BEGINS TO SHRINK

After taking the Cellfood she began to wake up in a sweat at night. Heat is what shrinks the tumor. After months of reporting that the tumor had stayed exactly the same size, she was delighted to tell me two months later on November 15, 2002, that it was harder and smaller! She said that the next week she would be working on the West Side of town where there is a good YMCA and would spend time working with weights, swimming, and doing the sauna. She was determined to meet her first deadline and be free of the tumor by Thanksgiving! She is willing to extend the deadline until the first of the year.

As a physician, Dr. Privitera is a very unusual and courageous man. He practices Alternative Medicine in California, a state bucking alternative methods of healing Cancer. The FDA, a government agency that is supposed to protect us, is actually a fierce guardian of the Economics of Conventional Medicine. They don't want the competition of any Doctors that prescribe vitamins and other natural means for Cancer. The main reason for their objections is entirely economic—if there are inexpensive, natural ways to get well from Cancer that work, the multi-billion dollar Cancer Industry would crumble! And they mean business!

"You have to fight," Dr. Privitera explains. "If you see the way to get well is by using natural alternatives, then you have to have the courage of your convictions!"

"You see, it is not the Cancer that kills the victim. It's the breakdown of the defense mechanism that eventually brings death. It is utter nonsense to claim that catching symptoms early and using "standard" medical treatment—surgery, chemotherapy, and radiation, will increase the patient's chances of survival. Not one Medical scientist or study has shown that," Dr. Privitera states.

LIVING LONGER WITH NO MEDICAL TREATMENT

Hardin Jones, a Berkeley Radiologist, decided after years of treating Cancer patients that "it did not matter if my machine was turned on or not!" He quit his Radiology job and went around the world doing research. To his amazement, after compiling his statistics, he found that if a person with Cancer did the Medical Treatment they lived an average of three years. A person with Cancer who did **nothing** at all lived twelve years!

It's time to wake up to the reality of what Cancer truly is. Cancer is a systemic, degenerative disease that cannot be cut, poisoned, or radiated out of the body. True health can only be reclaimed by empowering the immune system, changing the diet, adding vitamins and herbs, exercising, doing visualization, prayer, chanting, meditation, and changing our life to health enhancing routines, relationships, and environments. Experiments to inject Cancer cells into a healthy body fail to yield any negative results. Cancer cells do not have one iota of chance of existing or perpetuating themselves in the body of a strong, well nourished, internally clean, happy person!

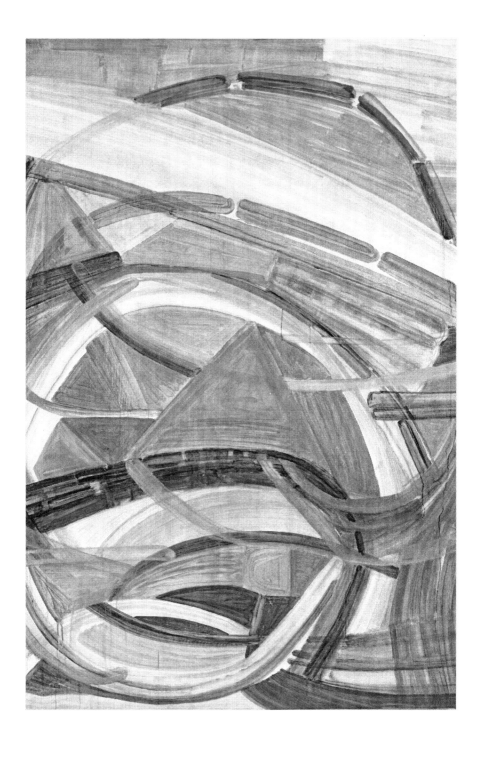

CHAPTER 7

Pathways to Healing

KARI DESCRIBED HER typical day on the MOTEP program with additional healing modalities. She was putting a lot of her effort and energy into restoring her health.

"I get up at six a.m. and do forty-five minutes of Wu Ming Meridian Therapy Qigong Movements."

She describes this as a Taoist Healing Center's methods of getting stagnating meridians moving. They have a book and a tape available at their New York center. They call this their Breast Cancer project and can be found on the web at BreastCancer.com. She does kicks and arm exercises such as "scooping the moon from the ocean, and opening curtains to let the Dragon in." All these exercises involve the arms and legs in vigorous motions.

"I then jump fifteen minutes on the rebounder, finishing off with twenty jumps with arms in the air affirming, I will win over Breast Cancer today."

She then drinks a glass of water with Cell-Food to create additional oxygen in her cells.

"After that I spend ten-to-fifteen minutes lying on the wood floor with a book under my head and rub a half-cut lemon, flaxseed oil, or apple cider vinegar on my lump. Lemon for the Vitamin C, flaxseed oil for the Vitamin E, Omega Three and Laetrile, and apple cider vinegar to kill parasites. I combine this with visualization, "seeing" the lump, starving, shrinking and disappearing.

"I then take my supplements with lemon water and green drink and make and drink a flaxseed smoothie. After getting dressed, I pray. Then I go to work."

Kari worked at a mortgage-lending firm. She did not get along well with her boss who had a bad temper and caused her a lot of distress. She reported to me joyfully one day that she found a way to move on, doing free-lance appraisals and will be able to obtain her license to freelance in six months. "I am ecstatic," she reports. "Now I feel like getting up in the morning!"

She comes home for lunch, her major meal. "I fix a salad, brown rice or barley, and a tofu burger or veggie burger. Or I might have salmon. Another day I might eat soybeans and lightly steamed vegetables."

She then goes to back to work. She snacks on dried apricots and apricot kernels, careful not to eat more than ten kernels a day. (I recommend no more than four.) However, Kari seems to assimilate the natural form of chemotherapy, vitamin B-17 that apricot kernels are loaded with, quite well. She also drinks plenty of spring water.

After work she goes home and jumps on the rebounder for fifteen minutes, finishing off with 120 jumps while affirming, "I have won over Breast Cancer today." She then goes for a forty-five minute power-walk with lots of arm movements affirming, "I have won over Breast Cancer today." Or she might say, "God, my immune system and I have healed the Breast Cancer." The arm movements, such as she would do swimming the breast stroke, back crawl, or rolling her arms while stretched out sideways or inward, bent at the elbows, rotating her fists, are very important in oxygenating her breast tissues. Oxygen kills Cancer cells. Cancer cells simply cannot live in an oxygenated environment.

After her walk, she juices carrots and other vegetables such as Collard Greens and beets, and eats steamed green beans, squash, or other vegetables with barley, or rice with tamari. "My big meal is lunch," she says. Before going to bed she re-reads *Keep Your Breasts*! for inspiration.

Kari lives with Rob, a younger man who she finds very compatible. She has gone through many relationships that didn't work out. Now she is happy and comfortable. He is anxious about her Breast Cancer and had a hard time being supportive of her natural program at first, however. She had to reassure him and her relatives that she is entirely confident she will get totally well. Every pioneer must face opposition. She is strong and determined. "I've changed my life!" she tells me joyously. Her destructive treatment of her body has given way to all-out, energetic nurturing and total support. "I feel great!"

YOU CAN CHANGE YOUR LIFE

I think it is just a matter of time before she will totally win over her disease. The day before Thanksgiving she reported to me that the lump is shrinking quite nicely after she began having shooting pains in her breast. This can be a sign of healing. Her boyfriend and relatives, following closely her progress, have come around. "It makes sense to build your health back up," they say, seeing the vast improvement in Kari's appearance. More about Kari's fight will be included later, even though she already feels victorious now.

AVA CONQUERS LEUKEMIA

At a garage sale one morning where I was looking for a cookie jar to hold my organic honey- sweetened cookies I made for the Art Walk, I encountered Verner who had a story to tell about her mother. She had been diagnosed with life-threatening Leukemia when she was only thirty-eight in 1955. Ava Macarthur was so sick she could not get out of bed and spent days crying, a weak and frail invalid.

Ava got sick over the years of distress she had experienced in her life. Her husband had a violent temper and hit her often. Verner and her brother and sister also got beaten. Ava, besides raising three children, also had to work every day, taking the bus to other people's homes to clean them. "It's the only work she knew how to do," Verna sighed. Taking care of three children with an abusive husband and cleaning homes became just too much stress for her. Eventually, her health broke down.

Ava had yellow skin and could hardly move. She had no energy at all. She became black around her eyes. She was deathly ill and failing fast. Everyone was certain she was on her deathbed. Finally, a woman at church urged her to see a Doctor Buchanan who treated Cancer holistically.

Dr. Buchanan, a medical doctor who practiced Alternative Medicine before it was fashionable, diagnosed her Leukemia but decided not to break the news until he had begun to restore her strength, which he did mainly with diet.

He told her that the blood gets so bad it becomes impossible to function normally as a person. To build her blood back, he put her on beets to build red blood cells. He had her boil this iron-rich vegetable and told her to also drink the water after they were cooked. To make this broth palatable, he suggested adding fresh pineapple juice to sweeten it. He had her eat mashed bananas topped with a mixture of rice polish, wheat germ and flax -seed.

"What is rice polish?" I asked Verna.

"It's what they polish and remove from brown rice to make worthless white rice. You see the 'dirty' part of the rice has all the B-vitamins. Under stress, you burn these vitamins quickly and become deficient. You can get rice polish at the health food store."

The doctor also gave Ava Vitamin B, C and calcium supplements. She was no longer to combine meat with starch such as potatoes. The diet he recommended emphasized vegetables and fruits. If she wanted meat she was limited to fish or chicken and only small amounts eaten with only vegetables. Also banned were lactic and citric combinations and no starches with fruits. No processed foods such as white sugar or white flour where allowed. Processed salt was also banned and sea salt recommended. " These processed foods are bleached which kills all the vitamin content," she told me. "When you strip the B-Vitamins from foods, people and animals die."

"A test for vitamin pills is to put them in a glass of water with one teaspoon of apple-cider vinegar," she said. "If they don't dissolve in twenty minutes, they are worthless." She remarked that a popular brand of vitamins is found still whole in people's stools. "It's important to get food-based vitamins," she said.

"Drugs only cover up the problems," Verna pointed out. "The body will respond to nourishment and vitamins. Then the immune system will take over and the problems will ease up and finally vanish."

"My mother lived in fear of her husband," she confessed. "When you worry and don't eat right, your body will break down."

The violence escalated until the police were called. "They did nothing. At that time, domestic violence was overlooked and disregarded. Calling the police only made Ava's husband more violent and viscious. Once he knocked me out cold."

Finally her father moved out. "He left my mother for another woman. I was only fourteen at the time. But it was a relief." Her mother got the small house and half his pension. Most important, however, was the peace of mind Ava was able to regain.

Dr. Buchanan slowly brought her mother back to health with his restorative diet. As an alternative practitioner before his time, he finally was kicked out and had to move his practice to Mexico.

It took Ava six-to-eight months to recover her zest for life, Verna remembered. "She began laughing again. She became more like her old self. It took her a year and a half to fully recover. She credits the diet, rest, prayer, and the loss of her abusive husband to her full and complete recovery. This was a real healing, not a remission," Verner pointed out. "She never in her life got Leukemia ever again."

"I'm glad I'm still alive," her Mother said the other day at age eighty-six.

"I don't eat sugar if I can avoid it." Verna remarked. "If I slip, I take alfalfa and garlic to help detoxify the toxins. I also like chicken broth, lots of lettuce and mustard instead of fats on my sandwich. I never get sick, not even colds or flu. When you eat whole foods instead of worthless processed ones, your body has the nutrients to stay well."

I always learn new health tips from the stories of long-term survivors of Cancer. I share their joy at beating the odds and amazing their conventional doctors, many of whom are not interested in what they did to accomplish their triumph. There is simply no money in it for them. Natural healing, though it provides a healing solution, rather than a temporary remission, and even though it saves lives, is a threat to their economic interests.

I CHANGED MY LIFE

My own story is just as miraculous. I decided I was willing to change anything and everything in order to save my own life. Because I was depressed over a failed relationship, had financial problems, and felt hopeless about my situation, I let my good health habits slip. But when Dr. Furr discovered the two tumors, I knew I had to turn my life around.

Eighteen years have gone by since I was diagnosed with both Breast and Uterine Cancer. No tumors have ever showed up again. I'm still on my MOTEP health program and have been free of Cancer and tumors for over eighteen years. After coming close to death, I have learned that the body and mind need care and attention, that the sacrifices and time one must take to preserve one's health are so crucial to longevity and happiness, they cannot be ignored. I have learned that being in harmony with one's environment, eating mostly organic fruits, vegetables, and whole grains, regular prayer and chanting, working hard but not worrying and fretting about the results, a regular, vigorous exercise program, and keeping my weight as close to my ideal as possible has paid off in happiness, health, and yes, even, success. My self-destructive drives have melted away in the mending of relationships, and sincere wish to help others and to give to others generously. I've turned my own life around and now help others to do the same.

It was a cold December day when my gynecologist found two tumors in my body, one in my left breast and one in my uterus. I had Cancer; in short order I would be fighting for my life. I was frightened into, not surgery as he insisted, but instead, a vigorous health program in which I determined to heal myself. Compiling the MOTEP health program, and going on it met with miraculous success. If I amazed my Gynecologist who was so aghast he joined the YMCA himself, I truly was the one most astonished at the ability of the body to rid itself of hard tumors that seemed like permanent rocks in just under two months! And though it did take seven more months to get well, I believed that supporting the body would eventually pay off in total health. As it did.

The first step one must take in this program is to detoxify the body and mind. This is done with a juicer, a blender, a detoxifying diet, a high-energy exercise program, and a spiritual program of prayer, meditation, and chanting in order to create a feeling of peace within the body. Only with a cleansed body, cleared of excess fats and toxins and a cleared mind, cleansed of anger, jealousy, resentment and other toxic, negative feelings, can the healing processes be jump-started. Cleaning the body internally takes a month to two months, depending on the amount of toxins and excess fats to be eliminated. Cleansing the mind takes as long as needed to get rid of these negative feelings and find the joy and peace in your life to replace them.

Once these two conditions have been met, supported by a vigorous exercise program of at least one hour per day, the healing processes will kick in. *In fact healing begins the very minute or second you decide to get well.* In my own case, the intense detoxification and de-stress program took one month. After a month, I was ready to go into the healing reaction. I don't like to call it the "healing crisis" although it was bad enough and terrifying enough to be called a crisis, the usual term for it. Healing reaction sounds more reassuring. But, still, it was extremely traumatic.

HEALING REACTION

The night before my reaction, I had a dream that my breast was rotting, turning yellow-green and disappearing and it stunk! It was the worst smell I had ever experienced. When I awoke, I still smelled that horrendous odor! It was then I was shocked into the realization that this was for real; my breast was actually beginning to rot! This is the bottom-line in Breast Cancer. Though no one ever talks about it. As the breast cells die off, they emit the putrid, rotting smell of death.

I was in a cold sweat! I had successfully detoxified my body for one month with freshly made orange juice in the morning and carrot juice in the evening, whole grains like barley and brown rice, and lots of fresh fruits and vegetables with only some fish for added protein. I had cut out all meat and dairy products and had under-eaten in calories while emphasizing many important nutrients. I had rubbed my breast with half-cut lemon morning and evening, alternating the next day with flax- seed oil. I had chosen to swim one mile five days a week and do the sauna before and after. I had even added half an hour of weights, machines and sit-ups before swimming. I chanted for twenty minutes morning and evening. I did visualization, "seeing" a scud missile hitting the tumor in the water while I swam and "watching" particles of it float off in the water. In the sauna, which I did before and after swimming, I visualized the rock in my breast melting like butter. Even though my financial situation was still perilous, and we were in the midst of the Gulf war with nothing on TV but scud-missiles loudly exploding and other destruction, I had somehow managed to overcome my fears and established a feeling of peace and well being in myself that I knew were absolutely essential for healing.

Now my body was ready. I went to the YMCA despite my fears and horrendous condition, and looked in the mirror in the locker room. I got the shock of my life! My left breast had turned a burning-neon red, was swollen, hard as a rock and hot to the touch. My left arm was inflated to three times its normal size and was totally paralyzed! I could not move it at all. It reminded me of a concrete freeway post! I have never been paralyzed in my life; I had somehow skipped the Polio epidemic. This was so traumatic I had trouble accepting that this was actually happening to me!

I decided to go swimming anyway. Other women would probably have panicked and called 911 and had an ambulance take them to a hospital. But I had total faith in the body's ability to heal itself, I reminded myself. Was this some carnival madness my body was going through—this hideous, grotesque display, in order to heal itself? Or was I dying? Was this part of the disease, a new disease, or a way of healing? I didn't really know.

So I swam using only one arm. As a teenage lifeguard, I had had a boss who had lost an arm in the war. I used to imitate him swimming with his one arm. He was a very strong swimmer. I had watched him go for miles that way, with his limitation. Now I had the same handicap. After about half a mile, I could get my left arm out of the water and throw it forward like a chunk of cement or a plywood board! I kept working it through. I was determined not to be permanently paralyzed!

This grotesque "healing reaction" for me only lasted one day. For others since, some have gone in and out of it for several months before they get well. But my body is very strong. I exercised most all of my life. As a teenager, I went on a salad diet, instead of the German meat-and-potatoes fare my Mother usually served. I was a swimmer and a skier; I hiked and camped out. All my life I have been athletic. Being a painter of large-scale canvases kept me in shape, lugging them around. I also jogged around a track at the local college before swimming in their large pool. I've never in my life been as much as ten pounds overweight. If I gain a few pounds, I take them off very soon if not immediately.

Yet it only took less than two years of serious depression with its subsequent loss of energy to exercise, overeating meat to try to compensate, filling my empty void with food, to lose my precious health, slowly becoming a very sickly person. A person with advanced Cancer. Two tumors and fading rapidly. A frightful looking version of my once healthful self greeted me upon looking in the mirror!

Yet, I was so very fortunate! With past healing experience and no health insurance to hypnotize me into believing that "they could get it all," I was under the gun to self-heal. Watching my friend Kimberly go through the Medical Treatment for her Breast Cancer was actually the greatest incentive not to get caught up with this mutilating and destructive version of "care."

When I watched the destruction of her body through the amputation of her lovely breast only to be stunned by the news that the Cancer had grown back in the very *same* spot—the chest wall where her breast used to be—I woke up. I suddenly realized that disease **cannot be cut out of the body!** It was then I began to come to grips with the reality that this fantasy, far from being "scientific," was only wishful thinking and profit-driven.

Later I found out that "loco-regional recurrence" of Cancer is quite common, sometimes as much as a third of all cases. ***Kimberly's Cancer growing back in the same spot where her breast used to be is not unusual.***

No, Cancer is never "local" and no, the tumor is **not** the disease. Since Cancer is a disease where a tumor often forms, cutting the tumor out is a simplistic and misinformed idea. That this would, necessarily, lead to a "cure," when in fact it is no more of a "cure" than cutting off the pox of a person with Chicken Pox, seemed suddenly extremely apparent to me. *A sick person needs to get well.*

NO "CURE" BUT WE CAN HEAL

Cancer is a systemic disease from the very beginning. It has to be healed from the inside out. Running or walking for a "cure" might be good exercise and a great fund-raising tool, but looking for this elusive "cure" may be wishful thinking. The reality is we must heal; we must get well. This can be done naturally with patience and effort, with supporting our immune system instead of destroying it with mutilation and poisons now called "therapies." Chemotherapy destroys the bone marrow where the blood cells are produced, creates gastrointestinal damage, renal failure, heart damage, brain damage, mouth sores, metabolic disorders, osteoporosis and long-term fatigue as well as secondary Cancers such as Leukemias. Secondary Primary Cancers are caused by dangerous radiation. Why would anyone submit to these toxins in the belief it would help them? After I saw Cancer could be healed using natural means to totally support the immune and healing systems, conventional Cancer treatment began to look suspiciously criminal. Large financial gain seemed far more important than the precious health of the patient!

"It makes sense," Kari told me. "Why should Cancer be treated with mutilation, dangerous surgery which explodes the tumor into leaking its cells to spread? Why use poisons in the deluded belief they will make you well?" She is now a convert, seeing her body gaining strength each day from the diet and exercise, the supplements and new career direction in her life, the visualization and good relationship she has developed with her younger boyfriend. Her tumor is definitely smaller, hardening and shrinking after three months of hard work. She is willing to be patient to be able to see it go away completely. Every day she sees her efforts pay off in a happier, healthier, more vigorous life.

Kari now has a new job she loves. "It gives me the emotional support to feel like getting well," she explains. She realizes the importance of her outlook on life.

Usually, Happy people don't get Cancer, is a Medical Maxim, I found, to my surprise in the Medical Literature when I did my research for my first book on Cancer. When people are happy, they don't destroy their bodies with negative habits and feelings such as anger, resentment, jealousy, grudges and other immune-suppressing emotions.

Kari became a pioneer. You can be one too!

CHAPTER 8

The MOTEP Healing and Prevention Diet

OF THE UTMOST importance, diet plays a crucial and pivotal role in the MOTEP healing program. This diet is a detoxifying diet, for the first step in healing in any Cancer is to rid the body of as much toxic material, excess fat content, clogged waste material, and stress hormones, such as excess estrogen, as possible.

Throughout history, thousands of people have healed their Cancer mainly through dietary means. Although I believe that the psychological aspects of Cancer are also crucial, diet is a pivotal factor in any healing. Changing the blood, cleansing it, and turning it back to normal composition takes work, but diet, vitamins, and herbs are powerful nutrients capable of restoring health. Miraculously, not only Cancer, but also other physical problems will begin to heal when the body is treated to a nurturing diet. Hippocrates, the Father of Medicine, said, "Let food be thy medicine and medicine be thy food." Hippocrates prohibited surgery in Cancer treatment, believing it too traumatic on the body and not effective at preventing recurrence.

The key to cleaning the body internally and still giving it super-nutrition is to concentrate on fresh fruits and vegetables, juicing, whole grains, fish, nuts, beans, and seeds. I also suggest under-eating for a month. The combination of eliminating meat and dairy products and utilizing whole grains helps remove excess fat and subsequent overproduction of estrogen that fat cells produce and/or store that often fuels Cancer growth. Breast Cancer, for instance, is often tested for estrogen receptors, the Cancer cells utilize for their development.

Under-eating also gives the immune system more room to move in to destroy tumors. A study that came out in April, 2003,[1] links obesity and overweight to Cancer. In fact ninety thousand deaths from Cancer are now attributed to obesity. As sixty-five percent of Americans are either overweight or obese, overeating now competes with smoking tobacco as one of the top factors in Cancer incidence.

In the study, men in the highest weight groups were fifty-two percent more likely to die from Cancer than those of normal weight, while women in the highest weight groups were sixty-two percent more likely to die from this insidious disease. Participants were drawn from over one million volunteers enrolled in the Cancer Prevention Program begun in 1982. The heaviest women died from Uterine, Kidney, Cervical, Breast, Gallbladder, Pancreas and Esophageal Cancers. Men died from Liver, Gall bladder, Stomach, and Colorectal Cancers. The few Cancers not found to be related to excess weight were brain, bladder, and skin Cancers.

Therefore losing excess weight is an important tool in Cancer healing. Simply by under-eating for a month will signal your body, if it has excess fat, to begin to clean out and

---

1 New England Journal of Medicine, April 24, 2003

release it. The following diet will help you do just that. In addition, the super-nutrition will help the body to destroy Cancer cells. A lean and mean body is what we are aiming for. How many obese old people do you see?

Though this diet was originally based on Michio Kushi's "Macrobiotic Diet," it has been enriched and expanded. Very few Western-raised people can thrive on such a minimal diet as Oriental people consume. Most Americans grew up on a meat and potato fare with lots of dairy products, and changing this diet takes a tremendous turn-around effort. Cancer is a signal to do just that.

The benefit of changing a saturated fat diet to a plant-based nutrition will show up in health, longevity, and a better looking body, clear eyes, and lack of health complaints. It's worth the effort, isn't it, to feel and look better? To have more energy and enthusiasm for life, get rid of cellulite and flab, pot-bellies, cellulite, acne, tooth-decay, bleeding gums, diabetes, cardiovascular disease, arteriosclerosis, and other problems associated with a highly refined, sugar and fat laden diet, is well worth the effort it takes to change, don't you agree? When you see the benefits begin to accumulate, you will come to love this diet. Always try to purchase and eat organic food, when possible.

DETOXIFYING THE BODY

The goal of the first two months is to clean out the body thoroughly in order to mobilize the healing forces. Your immune system will work far more efficiently when the body is clean. This is not much different than cleaning the filter for your gas, oil, or air in your car, heater, dryer, or any other machine you use. You will notice sluggish performance and even dying of these machines when their filters are clogged. Most Americans know about taking a shower everyday, but few people pay attention to the internal cleanliness of their bodies. To prevent or heal Cancer, a thorough intestinal cleaning out is a first and very pivotal step toward total healing. Many alternative authorities believe that most diseases start in a clogged-up colon.

DAY ONE

To start out gradually, on Day One, eat what you normally consume for breakfast and lunch. However, skip dinner and eat only an apple. This, preferably organic, apple should be non-shiny, as super-shiny apples are now coated with carcinogenic acrylic "wax." Be sure to drink plenty of spring water throughout the day and evening.

This is an easy, modified fast. Relieved of the job of having to digest dinner and armed with the fiber of the apple, the body will be able to go around and begin to clean out toxins, heading them to the intestines and liver and finally to the bowel for elimination. The next day you will spend more time in the bathroom as your body cleans out. You will start to feel better, lighter, and more energetic. A clean body is more efficient, less sluggish, and much healthier.

THE MOTEP DIET
DAY TWO

Today you can start the MOTEP diet. This diet emphasizes juicing with both the blender and a vegetable juicer. A wok, a cake-rack for steaming, a rice-cooker, and a Chinese cleaver are handy implements for this diet. Also a spice-grinder is a wonderful addition.

An important aspect of this diet is juicing. Both fresh fruit and fresh vegetable juices are important for their vitamins and minerals. You can consume a larger quantity of fruits and vegetables by juicing them. Normally eating eight large carrots and then trying to digest them would be a hardship. But juicing eight large carrots creates an easily consumable and digestible form of beta-carotene. The body will get instant vitamins. Cancer patients have been found consistently to be low in Vitamins, especially Beta-Carotene, the B Vitamins, Vitamin C, Vitamin D and Vitamin E.

Breakfast

Beginning the day with lots of vitamin-packed fruits and juices is easy with this recipe:

SUSAN'S SUPER-SMOOTHIE

In a blender container combine:

- One cup of fresh squeezed oranges, or half oranges and half tangerines (about 4 citrus fruits).

- One nickel-sized piece of fresh Ginger root.

- Three cups of chopped fresh fruit. (Example: eight Tablespoons Cantaloupe, one Red Plum, One Red or Green Pear, two Black Figs, ten raspberries). Bananas are always good additions. In the summer, combine them with peaches, nec-tarines, apricots, mangoes, and/or blackberries. Always include berries when in season as they are rich in Vitamin B-17, a natural form of che-motherapy. Use fresh rather than frozen fruit, if possible. The one and only exception I make to fresh fruit is canned pumpkin puree. This makes a delicious winter smoothie combined with pears, berries, and perhaps a banana.

- One-half cup of Amazake (a rice-nut drink) and one-half cup soy or rice milk

- One-half tsp. Nutmeg, one-fourth tsp. Cloves, and thee-fourths tsp. Cinnamon.

- Blend for two minutes or until well blended.

- If you cannot find Amazake, you can substitute soy yogurt.

This fills a blender container about two or three inches from the top. Be sure and put the blender top on tight! I drink all but one cup of this in the morning, saving a glass in the refrigerator for later when I get home from work.

Combined with cooked Oatmeal with raisins or bananas, whole grain toast, whole grain bagel or roll, this makes a complete breakfast. Granola is good and fast. I also like four-grain cereal with flax, or a multi-grain cooked cereal with barley.

The idea here is to skip the saturated fat breakfasts such as bacon, sausage, and eggs with buttered white-bread toast. For the whole-grain toast, a sugarless jam or honey or nut-butter is great instead of high-fat butter.

Spices have healing properties. In the *Los Angeles Times* Health section (January 19, 04), it was revealed that "a little bit of cinnamon might spice up your health." This aromatic bark can lower blood sugar, triglycerides and cholesterol levels, as well as improve Insulin functioning. It may be better than Statin drugs for reducing risk of cardiovascular disease. This should get you started on your morning.

A mid-morning snack is appropriate, such as a banana, grapes, or other fruit with herb tea or mineral water.

Lunch

Lunch for this detox-diet is a salad that can include watercress (rich in Vitamin B-17), or red-leaf lettuce, shredded carrots, green onions, and some lightly steamed or parboiled green beans, asparagus, or zucchini. You can vary the vegetables you use. Cooked fresh beets, broccoli, cauliflower, Brussel sprouts, okra, lima beans, snow peas, red or green peppers, radishes, and cabbage are all wonderful additions. The cruciferous families of vegetables are rich in indoles, known Cancer-fighting nutrients and include cabbage, brussel sprouts, broccoli, kale, and kohlrabi. For protein, steamed salmon, fresh seared tuna, macadamia nuts, and/or hard-boiled eggs can be added.

For a dressing, use two tablespoons flax- seed oil (which should be refrigerated), one tablespoon balsamic vinegar, one tablespoon fresh lemon juice, and one clove of finely chopped garlic seasoned with ground black pepper and sea salt or a bit of fresh rosemary, parsley, tarragon, or dill. Herbs commonly used in the kitchen have powerful antioxidant activity that fight free radicals, unstable molecules, and help heal the body. Olive oil is also good to use; best to use Extra-Virgin.

Flaxseed oil is the most powerful Cancer-healing oil, containing a high amount of Omega-3 fatty acids, so if you currently are fighting Cancer, begin with that. Omega-3 fatty acids are also found in fish, walnuts, and hemp-oil. These acids are crucial to healing. Eating fish has been found to cut stroke risk, for instance, as they lower levels of HDL, blood fats linked to cardiovascular disease and to help keep blood from clotting.[2]

For dessert a piece of fruit or two will round out the meal. To make a delicious serving, cut the fruit up, mix in some chopped walnuts and drizzle with a little Amazake or maple syrup. You can also heat up mixed fruit to make a variety "applesauce." You might drink either mineral water or herb tea with this. If you need to sweeten the tea, use honey. I like to add a bit of soymilk to cool it off.

Dinner

Start dinner with fresh-juiced carrots. Use seven or eight large carrots. The addition of a garlic clove or piece of fresh ginger- root adds spice. If you don't like straight carrot juice, it can be cut with a stalk of celery or an apple. Freshly juiced carrots taste sweeter and better than store-bought carrot juice that has sat around for a while, and the vitamin-content will also be stronger. Try it. Sip it slowly. If you have Cancer, visualize this vitamin-rich juice healing your tumor

_____

2 *Los Angeles Times, Associated Press News,* Dec. 23, 2002

or high white-blood cell count. Beta-Carotene is one of Cancer's most healing nutrients. It is absolutely essential after a diagnosis of Cancer to get a juicer and begin to use it, if you don't have one already. Flooding your internal system with fresh vitamins will point you immediately in the direction of health.

Later on you can experiment with juicing other vegetables. There are many books with wonderful juice combinations such as *Bragg Healthy Lifestyle—Vital Living to 120*, by Paul C. and Patricia Bragg, Health Science, Box 7, Santa Barbara, Ca. 93102, www.bragg.com.

On page 99, for instance, she suggests beet, celery and alfalfa sprouts; cabbage, celery, and apple; cabbage, cucumber, celery, tomato, spinach and basil; carrot, celery, watercress, garlic, and wheat-grass; and carrot, celery, parsley, cabbage, onion and sweet basil, for instance. These are delicious, healthful and worth trying. See what you like, but try to stick to carrot for the first two-to-four months, until you start to get well.

On the second day you might like one of my barley recipes for dinner. These make enough for lunch the next day. I guarantee this will help you to detoxify your body. Barley is the great clean-out grain, an ancient healing food. Both barley and flax seed oil contain Laetrile (Vitamin B 17), a natural form of Chemotherapy. Some of these foods are: chick peas, lentils, lima beans, mung bean sprouts, cashews, alfalfa, and almonds. Laetrile is also called Amygdaline from the Greek word Amygdale, meaning almonds (see Appendix-A for other foods). I use Barley regularly to rid my body of the toxins I accumulate as an Artist. I am regularly exposed to cobalt, cadmium, lead and other dangerous metals in my paint as well as strong solvents. Yet, I am very healthy and have lots of energy!

Fresh Oregano has 42 times the Antioxidant activity of apples! Nuts also have Laetrile, but use them sparingly as they are high-calorie and fattening when overeaten. Tomatoes have Lycopine and especially when cooked, have shown to prevent and heal Prostate Cancer. Garlic and onions and their related cousins (scallions, leeks, and shallots) are part of the alum family and contain an important nutrient, Selenium. This nutrient is an ancient and known Cancer-healer. Garlic was used by the ancient Egyptians as a remedy for Cancer. In Japan, people who consumed scallions every day had less Cancer.

This recipe is adapted from *Food and Wine* Magazine.

MEDITERRANEAN ALMOND-BARLEY

- One-fourth cup almonds
- One-cup pearl barley
- Three tablespoons olive oil
- One medium onion, finely chopped
- Two large tomatoes, chopped
- Two garlic cloves, minced
- One-half teaspoon ground cumin
- One-half teaspoon ground coriander
- One-half teaspoon ground turmeric
- One bunch fresh oregano

1. In a medium saucepan, cover the barley with about three inches of water.
2. Add two tablespoons chopped oregano. Stir to blend. Bring to a boil. Cover and simmer over low heat until the barley has split and is tender but slightly chewy, about 35-40 minutes. Keep checking the water to make sure the barley doesn't stick and burn.
3. In a wok, heat two tablespoons of the oil. Add the almonds and stir-fry for two minutes. Pour off the nuts into a heavy container to cool. When cooled put nuts into a blender container and pulse twice to coarsely grind them.
4. Add one-tablespoon oil to wok. Add the onion and cook over moderate heat until tender, about three- to—five minutes. Add the tomatoes and cook until their juices thicken, about four minutes. Add the garlic and cook two more minutes until fragrant. Add the cumin, coriander, and two tablespoons more of the fresh oregano and cook another three minutes. Add the barley and one-cup spring water. Cover and simmer until flavors are nicely blended about four minutes. Season with fresh ground pepper and sea salt and serve with steamed vegetables such as green beans, okra, broccoli, or squash.

This is good cold, packed for lunch the next day also. You are on your way to cleaning out your body. You will notice you spend more time in the bathroom as your body does its Spring Cleaning!

DAY THREE

Start the day with "Susan's Super Smoothie." With it eat granola or cooked mult-grain cereal with soymilk or Amazake, and perhaps raisins or a banana.

Mid-morning snack can be red grapes.

Lunch is leftover Mediterranean Barley and two or three pieces of fresh fruit. Or have a freshly made vegetarian sandwich of dark whole-grain seeded bread spread with Dijon mustard, with a filling of avocado, tomato, spinach leaves, and sprouts. Some healing books are against eating leftovers, as they do not contain the energy or "Prana" of fresh foods. For me, eating parts of last night's dinner packed for studio lunch consumption is quick and easy. I still recovered from Cancer and have been totally well for eighteen years. You decide.

Dinner can be steamed salmon and vegetables and is quick and easy to make.

SIMPLE STEAMED SALMON WITH ROSEMARY:

- One salmon steak, washed off

- Two cloves garlic, chopped

- Two twigs fresh Rosemary

- Half-cut Lemon

  Vegetables:

- Green beans, zucchini, broccoli or wedge of cabbage

- Corn on the cob

Try to get wild-caught salmon instead of farm-raised salmon. Farmed salmon are given antibiotics, pesticides, and even food coloring to make them look pink! They also are kept in small cages so they don't get the exercise needed to develop their HDL, or healthy fats from swimming around. Omega-3 fats developed in wild fish are more abundant and necessary to heal Cancer. That's the main reason to eat fish! Taming and caging fish for eventual slaughter is repugnant to me!

Put a cake-rack in your wok and add water three-quarters of the way up to the rack. Heat the water. Prepare the fish by sprinkling it with garlic and Rosemary, and place on the rack alongside the vegetables and corn on the cob. Squeeze lemon over the fish. Sprinkle fish and vegetables with sea salt and fresh-ground pepper. Put the top on the wok and steam for about ten-to- fifteen minutes or until fish becomes a muted pink color inside. Remove Rosemary twigs and serve. Additional flaxseed oil can be added to the vegetables.

The addition of flaxseed oil to my diet, only one or two tablespoons per day, also rid me of allergies I have had since childhood! I used to sneeze seven-to-ten times in a row if I encountered perfume, cigarette smoke, smog, cold, or almost any aroma or temperature change. Now, I no longer react in this embarrassing and disruptive way. Also, I no longer get my yearly winter flu or colds. A bit of flaxseed oil everyday will be a tremendous boost to your health!

For a party, I steam a whole Salmon in the oven in a roasting pan. Raise the fish up a bit by putting it on a rack and add water. Cover the roasting pan with lid or foil and roast at 350 degrees for about half-an hour. Guests will ask you who cooked the salmon for you!

DAY FOUR

Start with Susan's Super Smoothie. Whole grain pancakes can be made with one egg. Maple syrup is fine to use. The sugar you need to avoid is refined, white sugar and artificial sugar-substitutes such as Nutri-Sweet that is carcinogenic. Brown sugar is no better as it is only refined sugar that has a bit of molasses added back.

Lunch

Lunch can be a spinach and red cabbage salad with left-over salmon or a hard- boiled egg. A piece or two of fruit and a few honey graham crackers make a nice dessert.

Dinner

A light soup supper can be made. Here is a suggested recipe:

MISO SOUP WITH WATERCRESS AND BROWN-RICE NOODLES

- Six cups spring water

- Four ounces noodles, preferably brown-rice noodles

- One clove garlic, chopped

- One Tsp. chopped fresh ginger root

- Two Tbs. olive oil

- Two Tablespoons miso, preferably made from barley

- One bunch watercress, chopped

- One box (12.3 ounces) firm tofu, cubed

- One large carrot, sliced on the diagonal

- One-fourth cup shelled English peas

- Two tablespoons fresh lime juice

- Two tablespoons tamari soy sauce

- One spring onion, sliced on the diagonal

Boil six cups water in a medium saucepan. Add noodles and cook stirring occasionally until al dente, about eight minutes. Drain.

Meanwhile in another medium saucepan, heat olive oil. Add garlic and ginger and cook stirring, about two minutes. Slowly and carefully add four cups of spring water. Stir. Add two tablespoons soft Miso and stir well. Add noodles, watercress, peas and carrots. Simmer five minutes. Add lime juice, cracked pepper and tamari soy sauce. Stir well. Top with chopped green onions, swirl, and ladle into soup bowls and serve.

Serves 3-4.

This tastes authentically Japanese, though I made up the recipe. The Japanese diet protects against Cancer. For instance, their Breast Cancer rate is one-eighth that of the U.S. when people eat the traditional Oriental diet.

If you want a dessert, melon is wonderful. Cantaloupe is very high in Beta-Carotene as is watermelon.

DAY FIVE
Breakfast

Start by making the smoothie. Prepare French toast with dark, whole grain, seeded bread and one egg mixed with one-fourth cup of soy- milk. You can use maple syrup on it. Or cook whole-grain cereal with raisins in spring water or soy- milk.

Lunch

Mid-day meal can be Miso soup from last night's dinner, reheated. Or make a tuna-salad sandwich in a whole-wheat pita bread. Eat two or three pieces of fruit for dessert. If you eat an apple, eat some of the seeds. These contain Laetrile, Vitamin B-17, Nature's chemotherapy.

Dinner

Pan grilled Tuna with Mustard Sauce and Zucchini, with Flax Fried Rice with Vegetables and Nuts is terrific and packed with Cancer-fighting nutrients.

FLAX FRIED RICE WITH VEGETABLES AND NUTS

- Two Tbs. Flaxseeds

- One cup cooked brown rice

- Two Tbs. Olive Oil

- Two cloves garlic

- One Stalk Celery

- Two green onions, chopped

- Juice of One-half lemon

- Two Tbs. Flax –seed oil

- One-Fourth cup Macadamia Nuts

Grind Flaxseeds fine in a spice-grinder. Heat a wok. Add olive oil. When hot add garlic and celery and stir-fry one minute. Add rice and stir-fry. Add flax- seed and stir-fry three minutes. Add green onions, lemon juice and macadamia nuts. Season with Sea Salt and fresh ground black pepper. Turn off heat. Drizzle with flaxseed oil.

PAN GRILLED TUNA WITH
MUSTARD SAUCE AND ZUCCHINI

- MUSTARD SAUCE

- Three tablespoons flaxseed Oil

- One clove garlic, minced

- One Tbs. Coarse Country Dijon Mustard

- Two pieces of thick, fresh tuna (about three-fourths pound)

- Two Tbs. olive oil

- One zucchini cut into coins

Make sauce by combining sauce ingredients in small bowl. Heat a cast-iron frying pan. When hot, add olive oil. When hot, add tuna to sear it. Cook two minutes. Turn to cook the other side two minutes. Spoon sauce over both tuna medallions. Add zucchini. Let zucchini brown two minutes, turning often. Season all with Sea Salt and Fresh Cracked Pepper. Put lid on pan, reduce heat to low, and cook for 5-8 minutes. Tuna will be rare at 5 minutes. Serve tuna with zucchini and rice. Serves two.

This dinner saved me from getting ill after a cold, dark, rainy day at the studio and running errands in the rain afterwards, getting soaked. For Cancer, this dinner is the ultimate in healing foods. Be sure each dinner to start with fresh carrot or carrot-celery juice. Kari recommends carrot-cilantro. For extra healing power, try carrot-garlic. Garlic was known in ancient Egypt as a remedy for Cancer.

After eating this dinner, take a glance in the mirror and see your color change to a richer hue!

Now you get the general idea of how to eat on this diet from the five-day plan. The American Cancer Society lists the following fruits and vegetables they feel contribute to preventing Cancer: apples, artichokes, red onions, bananas, strawberries, collard greens, papayas, lettuce, tomatoes, broccoli, oranges, potatoes, bell peppers, prunes, carrots, Swiss chard, spinach, apricots, avocados, acorn squash, Savoy cabbage, celery, cauliflower and sweet potatoes.

These are all worth incorporating into your diet.

I have a favorite Barley Recipe for another healing supper to share with you. I got the idea from the Pesto-pasta served at Little-Joe's in San Francisco where I stood in line on the sidewalk with my friends awaiting the wonderful, hot green dish. It was unforgettable! I've adapted it here using Barley for its healing properties. This recipe will make you feel great!

BRIGHT-GREEN PESTO BARLEY

- Two Tbs. olive oil

- One cup pearl barley

- Five cups spring water

- Two large bay leaves

- Sea salt and fresh ground black pepper

Pesto:
- Two tbs. chopped garlic

- One cup fresh basil leaves, chopped

- One-half cup fresh parsley, chopped

- One-half cup cashews

- One-fourth cup olive oil

- One-fourth cup boiling spring-water

- Juice of one-half Lemon

- Sea salt and fresh-ground pepper

In a large saucepan, heat the olive oil. Add barley and toast, stirring, about eight minutes until browned. Add bay leaves and boiling Spring- water. Cook forty-five minutes, stirring often until water is absorbed.

Combine Pesto ingredients in a blender-container. Blend until well combined and semi-liquid.

Discard bay leaves from barley. Add Pesto and stir well. Cook on low heat ten minutes, stirring. Add lemon juice and serve.

THE DETOX DIET

Now you get the idea and flow of this detox-diet. After a couple of months, along with the exercise program, the mental de-stress activities, and other principles of the MOTEP program, your immune system will be strengthened and encouraged to continue the healing process. This is a spare diet in which you under eat, but load your body with nutrients and fiber. When you get well, you can include a bit of chicken or other meat, but use sparingly. I stick to the Chinese way of eating by combining a bit of meat with lots of vegetables and rice. Don't eat large steaks or roasts, hamburgers, hot dogs, or large pieces of pork on a regular basis if you have had Cancer or are trying to get well from it. Vegetarians consistently show a lower Cancer risk. Meat is high in saturated fat, calorie dense, and hard to digest. The older you get, the harder it is to digest large chunks of meat. When invited out, if the hostess serves meat, you can eat a bit of it. Complaining and objecting is negativity. You want to praise the hostess.

This diet is not rigid. I eat just a bit of whatever is served, smile and find some compliment to give the host or hostess.

Eat lots of salads. In the summer, especially, I love a large salad of fresh, raw and lightly cooked vegetables for dinner. I use red-leaf, spinach, or romaine lettuce, shredded carrots, cooked beets, string beans, cucumbers, tomatoes, red or yellow peppers, green onions, and a dressing of flax-seed oil, lemon juice, grainy mustard, balsamic vinegar, minced fresh garlic, and a tiny bit of spring water. You can vary the vegetables according to what looks good at the Organic or Farmer's Market.

Supplements of Vitamin and Minerals should be added. I took a multi-vitamin and mineral capsule, as well as Vitamin B Complex, Vitamin C, and Vitamin E. The minerals that are important are Selenium, Magnesium, and Calcium. Echinacea is also good for stirring up the immune system. Melatonin, given to mice, slowed tumor growth. But mainly, rely on fresh, organic food.

For lowering cholesterol, diet could be as effective as drugs.[3]

University of Toronto researchers designed a diet with soy, vegetables, almonds and plant sterols (which block the absorption of cholesterol). Men and women ate only this diet for one month. Within two weeks, participants had reduced their low-density lipoprotein, or bad cholesterol by nearly thirty percent on average, maintaining it for the month.

"That's about the same reduction we see in people who take cholesterol-lowering drugs," says Dr. David J.A. Jenkins, professor of medicine and nutritional science.

Remember that unhealthy fats can clog the cells as well as the arteries. Fats that are bad for your health include margarine, solid vegetable shortening, and any oils commonly sold in grocery stores in clear bottles. These oils have been subjected to high-temperatures to improve their shelf life. Unfortunately the good vitamins have been heated out, and dangerous Trans-fats that clog arteries and cells have

---

3 *Los Angeles Times,* Monday, December 16, 2002, pp. F2 Health Section

been created. Stick to flax oil in dark bottles and extra virgin olive oil.

Eating this diet for two months will begin the healing process for any type of Cancer. You are on the healing path!

In Appendix B are suggestions for healthy cookbooks. However, you can convert any fat-laden recipe and even bake by substituting olive oil or flax-seed oil for butter, soy milk for cow's milk, and maple sugar, turbinado sugar, honey, molasses, maple syrup, or other natural sweeteners for white or brown sugar. And I always use whole grain flours packed in small bags and kept refrigerated.

I am now known as a healthy baker who can turn out a spectacular birthday cake that is also nutritious. For my friend Marion's birthday, I baked a Bundt cake using a mixture of whole-grain pastry flour and barley flour, honey, olive oil, and poppy-seeds as well as the usual eggs and other ingredients. When it came out of the oven, brown and lovely, I filled the hole with a mixture of fresh, organic strawberries and raspberries. Everyone thought I had stopped off at a bakery! This recipe was adapted from Deborah Madison's *Vegetarian Cooking for Everyone* (Broadway Books, N.Y.).

Healthy restaurants are easier to find now. Skip the steakhouse, the hamburger joint and the greasy spoon, and opt for Chinese, Thai, Japanese, California Fresh, Fish and Seafood restaurants and other health-oriented places. You can always order a salad and fish that is broiled, grilled, poached, or steamed instead of deep-fried. Bon appetite!

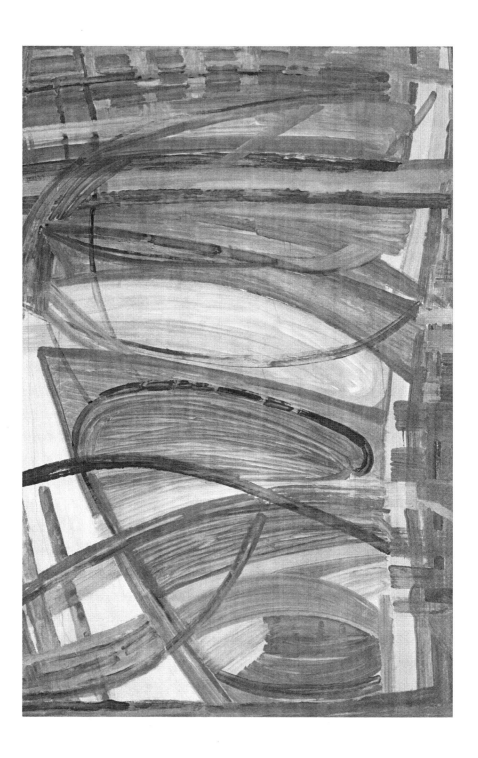

CHAPTER 9

On Your Mark, Get Ready, Get Set, Go! Leaping Into Health

THE SPRINGBOARD BACK to health from any Cancer is vigorous exercise. Also, the clearest route to prevention is aerobic exercise.

Kari called very excited on January fourth, 2003. She had been on the MOTEP program four months along with additional supplements prescribed by Dr. James Privatera whom she had visited a week ago. With her vigorous exercise program, not only has she been able to return her blood back to normal during the first month, she also was able to shrink her tumor by half. It has now taken on the characteristics of a benign fibroid lump!

This was news to me, as I never went through this transition. My tumors, with the help of swimming a mile five days a week, disappeared after a stunning heat-reaction in which my breast turned bright, neon red and became hard as a rock and hot as a stove. My left arm swelled to three times its normal size and became stiff and completely paralyzed. The massive lymph-fluid infusion was flooding and cleaning out the Cancer cells! After my swim that I did anyway with one arm this reaction slowly subsided. In about a day-and-a-half, my arm resumed its normal size. The breast and uterine tumors were in my body only one more week and then disappeared completely and haven't returned in eighteen years!

However, in Kari's case, her regression to a benign fibroid should be news to the Medical Establishment. This stunning development shows that fibroid lumps can advance to Cancerous tumors and Cancerous tumors can regress back to benign fibroid lumps! This was all achieved with exercise, nutrition, prayer, redirecting her life to a positive direction, good relationships, and topical natural treatments, without the utilization of any drugs, radiation, surgery or hormone treatments.

Kari swears by her re-bounder, a mini-trampoline, along with walking three miles with the addition of vigorous arm movements. She was such an avid jumper, vigorously using her arms at the same time that she went through, literally, one re-bounder in two months and had to buy a new one! She did this re-bounding for fifteen to twenty minutes morning and evening.

Kari met Dr. Morton Walker the author of *Jumping for Health—A Guide to Re-Bounding Aerobics* (Avery-Penguin-Putnam) at the Cancer Convention. According to Dr. Walker, re-bounding causes bone marrow to increase production of red blood cells, while sedentary bone marrow becomes lazy and inactive. Exercise in general has been found to make participants feel more alive and less tense. For Kari, the addition of vigorous arm movements helped oxygenate the tumor area, literally wiping out Cancer cells and creating an environment of healthy tissue in which Cancer cells will degenerate and disappear. While she did this vigorous exercise, she incorporated affirmations, such as "I am winning over Breast Cancer."

I incorporated visualization, as I am a visual artist and am able to "see" what does not exist. While I swam I visualized a scud missile hitting my tumor and "saw" white particles of it disperse into the water. Combining exercise with visualization and affirmations contributes a powerful healing tool for the body's Cancer fighting arsenal.

CELL OXYGENATION

By subjecting the sixty trillion cells in your body to high oxygenation and utilizing gravity that you work against when you jump, swim, lift weights, walk or row a boat, the cells are cleansed of waste products, damaged cells eliminated, and nutrition is drawn in. For healthy cells, oxygen is nutrition. For Cancer cells, oxygen is a wipe out eliminator. Regular exercise also increases metabolism and keeps it at its healthiest level.

Nathan Pritikin, famous for his books on health and diet advice, blamed the sedentary way of life inherent in our white collar occupations and spectator sports where we only sit and watch rather than participate, for failing to provide sufficient oxygenation of the body's cells. These cells can then break down and turn Cancerous.

In Colon Cancer, Dennis Burkitt, M.D., the noted British internist who first identified a malignancy called Burkitt's lymphoma, states that the deoxycholic acid and anaerobic excretion products formed when food is digested, lodge exactly at the site where Colon Cancer forms. With regular exercise, quantities of oxygen are infused into the blood stream to the colon. This creates an unfavorable environment for the growth of Cancer.

In Lung Cancer, often caused by inhaling cigarette smoke, asbestos, or other powders and dust such as sawdust or hairspray, exercise saturates the lungs with oxygen helping to counteract the damage, helping the cells to eliminate the dust or smoke, and cleansing the tissues.

HIGH CHOLESTEROL AND SMOKING

Jeremiah Stamler M.D. of Chicago's Board of Health tested nine hundred people for a relationship of the number of cigarettes they smoked and Lung Cancer. He couldn't find a relationship. However, he did find a connection between high cholesterol levels and Lung Cancer. If the serum cholesterol level was 275 milligrams percent or more, there were eight times as many cases. If the serum cholesterol level was below 150 milligrams, however, there was *no* Lung Cancer. High cholesterol not only blocks arteries, it contributes to the blocking of the white blood cells, such as macrophages that vacuum up Cancer cells by swallowing and digesting them.

With exercise and high-oxygenation, the chemistry of the blood is modified. Exercise increases the good fats (HDL) and decreases the bad ones (LDL). High-density lipoproteins (HDL) are part of the body's cleansing system, while Low Density Lipoproteins contribute to Cancer. These fats are also found in the diet when we ingest bad trans- fats like hydrogenated vegetable oils such as shortening and margarine, and processed, heat-treated oils found on most grocery shelves in clear bottles.

In a study by Methodist Hospital in Houston, Texas,[1] it was found that the more people routinely incorporated aerobic exercise into their daily schedule, such as re-bounding, running, bicycling, swimming, rope-skipping and vigorous walking, the higher their blood levels of HDL. These researchers stressed amount of exercise over what people ate. Very active exercises had as much as twenty parts higher of HDL in their blood as the inactive participants in the study.

Emotional benefits are also accrued with exercise. Psychologically, the empowerment and control it provides will strengthen the will to live and give the exerciser a positive frame of mind, reducing or eliminating depression. Cancer specialists who practice alternative medicine who are themselves risk-taking individualists, note that patients willing to participate in their own healing are a self-selected group. They need to take charge of their lives, not following the crowd. In oncology, unfortunately, following the crowd often means a tortuous death.

BUILD YOUR LIFE AROUND EXERCISE

Building your life around an exercise routine, rather than finding some time to exercise is a completely different concept. My first step on the MOTEP program after hearing my diagnosis of Breast and Uterine Cancer and deciding to take action rather than feel sorry for myself was to join the YMCA. *First you Cry,* a book on Breast Cancer by Betty Rollins, was changed to First you Exercise. You can rely on the often proven fact that oxygen kills Cancer cells. Cancer cells are anaerobic, and cannot exist or metastasize in a highly oxygenated environment.

---

1 *New England Journal of Medicine,* Feb.14, 1980

At the "Y" I spoke with Mike Cole telling him frankly that I had just been diagnosed with Stage Four Cancer and wanted him to help me to design an exercise program to recover my health. After consulting with him and thinking over my own past healing experience, I opted to swim a mile five days a week. Now I precede that mile with a half-hour of weights, sit-ups, and machines. To do all this, I get up at five in the morning. This may sound extreme, but there is a good-size group of people who do it at the "Y" and I simply join the early birds. Your body will soon acclimatize itself to a new schedule, whatever you devise. In the past, I exercised after work. I did an hour of aerobics with half-an-hour of swimming and sauna at the old Jack La Lannes' club. Remember him? He's still around at this writing, lifting his weights and swimming in the ocean bodily towing boats! "I can't die," he explains. "It would ruin my image!"

The principal at work here is that Cancer cells are anaerobic, meaning they thrive in an environment that lacks oxygen. The simple fact that oxygen kills Cancer cells is one you can take advantage of every time you engage in any exercise routine that increases your heart rate or uses your muscles. Intake of oxygen must match expenditure of energy by the muscles. That is, you will take in more oxygen the more you move!

Otto Warburg, a Nobel-prize winning scientist, showed in an often-duplicated experiment that normal cells can be turned into Cancer cells merely by depriving them of oxygen! The Nobel Prize winner insists that the real cause that stimulates a single cell to start subdividing spontaneously, quickly, and without a discernable pattern to its mitosis is the lack of oxygen at the cellular level. When oxygen starvation because of tensed posture; stressed, shortened breathing habits; sedentary lifestyle; and/or oxygen depriving exposure to cigarette smoke or other fumes or dust in the environment, cells turn from respiration to fermentation in order to obtain their energy. These cells thrive on sugar. Thus combining many hours of watching TV, driving, and sitting down at work, to eat, to watch sports or movie, with a highly refined sugar and saturated fat diet creates the most conducive lifestyle for Cancer growth! Does this sound like the average American lifestyle?

The body needs a plentiful supply of oxygen to defend itself against disease, eliminate waste products, repair damaged tissues and cells, and regenerate new ones. Since we now know one of he prime causes of Cancer is lack of oxygenation of the cells, it is only common sense to incorporate an aerobic exercise program into your daily life.

BLOOD CHEMISTRY

James H. Jandl in his *Textbook of Hematology* notes that "Neoplastic (Cancerous cell) populations are not programmed to complete normal cell differentiation; they fail to mature and gather in unfinished, undirected bewilderment."

He also states that slow-growing Cancer cells respond poorly to chemotherapy. Rather than poison them, why not oxygenate them to disable them? Oxygen is a much more permanent solution to wiping out Cancer cells than chemotherapy, which is almost always a temporary and very physically damaging "solution." Chemotherapy destroys the immune system's white blood cells, giving Cancer cells free rein to proliferate rapidly and spread at a dramatic rate. Cut them off at the pass with a high-dose of self-propelled oxygen!

These cells are confused and need direction. Give that to them with aerobic exercise combined with affirmations and visualizations. Be firm with these wayward cells! See your cells gaining direction and control as you exercise. See them gain strength and health. *They will respond when you are not confused or ambivalent about getting healthy again, but are able to give them strong direction.*

SEDENTARY LIFESTYLE

The sedentary lifestyle is the culprit in many cases of overweight and obesity in both children and adults. When people worked hard in the fields all day at the beginning of the century, with no TV, few automobiles, Video games, fast-food restaurants, computers, and other "labor-saving" devices, Cancer was a rare disease. People got up early and did a lot of hard, physical labor, often outdoors in clear, fresh air and warming sun. They walked to places they wanted to go. Spare time was often spent in participating in sports activities rather than watching them on the tube. People spent most of their day energetically moving around.

Today people get in the car, then onto an escalator or elevator, in order to sit for hours at a desk!

Now that over a quarter of our children are overweight or obese, and sixty percent of our adult population need to lose weight, Cancer is an epidemic!

EARLY RESEARCHER ON EXERCISE AND Cancer

James Ewing (1866-1943) was an early Cancer researcher who discovered the benefits of exercise as an avoidance measure of Cancer. In 1920 he did a study of eighty-six thousand Cancer patients; the results revealed the highest death rate among those that did the least exercise.

In 1931 he gave a series of Belmont Lectures entitled, "Causation, Diagnosis and Treatment of Cancer." He pointed out that Cancer was the most difficult subject in Modern medicine and that the average physician in Massachusetts sees two cases a year! (Some states were lower)!

I wonder what he would think of the one-out-of two men and one-out-of-three women rate of Cancer in 2008! He worried about the failure of the multitudinous efforts to find a cure for Cancer. But he stated, *"It is a serious and popular misconception that Cancer is a great mystery."* Also he believed it was a fantasy and waste of time to try to find an "overnight cure." Cancer entails a complex healing process, he pointed out.

"While we ignore the causation and frantically look for some new discovery that will put us in control of malignant tissue," he stated, "finding the cure for Cancer is not hopeful." He also pointed out that tissues react to injury by inflammation and regeneration.

In my own experience of healing, this is exactly what happens in Cancer healing. The body uses heat and inflammation, creating warmth and redness, a "fever" in the tumor area. In the Medical terminology, Breast Cancer that shows these symptoms is known as "Inflammatory Breast Cancer," considered as the most dangerous and threatening form of

Cancer with a two-percent survival and an eighteen-month or-less mortality prognosis. However, I found this dramatic process to be the "healing reaction" or healing crisis my body went through in order to rid itself of disease. This misconception, I believe, is at the root of our failure to stem the tide of escalation in Breast Cancer mortality. *We don't understand and refuse to learn how the body itself heals Cancer.* Yet with an all-natural program of support including vigorous exercise, the body is fully capable of healing Cancer and returning the body back to full and robust health. *Once this is accomplished, the threat of recurrence is greatly diminished.*

USING THE SAUNA TO HEAL

Heating the body to induce healing by sitting in a sauna before and after exercising is an essential part of the MOTEP exercise program. American Indians utilized "sweat lodges" in which high-heat was used to as a healing and spiritual environment for the tribe's illnesses.

James Ewing points out that the Ancients did not use Surgery for Cancer treatment. They used heat to help bring on the inflammatory reaction. Removal by knife became the vogue after anesthesia was discovered. By knocking out a woman, a Radical Breast Amputation could more easily be performed.

(I like this nomenclature, which is more descriptive than "Mastectomy.") Originally mastectomies were done without any anesthesia!

He found that the results from "Radical Breast Amputations" with the dissecting of supraclavicular and other lymph nodes were not satisfactory. The extensive operation in which they took out not only the breast, but also the chest muscles, sawed into the clavicle (collarbone) to remove lymph nodes as well as axillary or under-arm lymph nodes, resulted in high mortality rate from the operation itself! He found radiation also unsatisfactory as many tumors are not radiosensitive and radiation resulted in slow-growing secondary Cancers that would appear sometimes twelve years or more later.

The mutilating "Radical Breast Amputation" resulted, at best, with three-year "cures," he noted, while there were *no* survivors after ten years! No insurance company at that time accepted this operation because of this dismal life expectancy! (How times have changed!)

Dr. Ewing, who Ewing's Sarcoma was named after—Sarcomas are malignant tumors that begin in connective tissues, not Epithelial, (skin, mouth, larynx or urinary bladder)—believed that what was actually needed in Cancer was to *eliminate the causes*. He recommended rest, relief from the irritation that may have caused it (pipe or cigarette smoking, working with carcinogenic materials, exposure to radioactive materials), increased exercise, and nutrition. He observed that Cancer was highly susceptible to mental suggestion, thus paving the way for researchers to hone in on why psychological factors influence the growth of Cancer.

He ends his lecture pointing out that Rohdenberg collected three-hundred- forty-six cases of spontaneous regression, (the complete disappearance of Cancer naturally without treatment), and this represented a higher number of survivors than all the Cancer cures put together! Later in 1966 Everson and Cole published *Spontaneous Regression of Cancer* detailing two hundred cases of Cancer that suddenly, almost magically, disappeared without medical treatment.

Exercise, I believe, was the jump-start my body needed for its "spontaneous regression" of two tumors.

VISUALIZATION AND EXERCISE

Dr. O.Carl Simonton with Stephanie Matthew Simonton who invented visualization and describe how to do it in their book, *Getting Well Again* state, "We began paying more attention to exercise when we discovered that many of our patients with the most dramatic recoveries from Cancer were physically very active." The reasons they found exercise works to heal Cancer is that it releases stress and tension, changes one's state of mind, and gave their patients a way to actively participate in their own healing.

Aerobic exercise in which you pant and sweat raises the temperature of the body, giving it the heat it needs to heal. At the same time you are taking in the oxygen needed to wipe out Cancer cells and nourish and strengthen the normal cells. Further, exercise stimulates the immune system, revitalizes the organs, increases blood flow, increases the metabolic rate so that toxins are eliminated (also they are eliminated through the sweat glands), and lowers the fat content of the body. You are changing the chemical composition of the body making it more favorable to normal cells and inhospitable to Cancerous ones.

In devising your exercise program, keep in mind the following requirements:

1. Pick an aerobic Cardiovascular exercise that will involve large muscle groups, increase the heart rate, and demand for oxygen

2. Choose one that pits your muscles against a resistance or workload such as weights, water, or gravity.

3. Gravitate toward one you will enjoy doing approximately one hour a day, five-to-six days a week.

4. Go for one that that will decrease the fat-to-lean ratio of your body. Healing takes place faster in a lean-and-mean and clean body.

5. Choose one that will let you "space-out," do affirmations and visualizations while exercising thus creating a psychologically healing environment while enjoying a physically healing one. Recent research at the University of Illinois has compared MRIs of the brain of those physically fit and athletic to those who are sedentary. Researchers found that the brain keeps more brain tissue in the physically active compared to more deterioration of brain tissue in the sedentary.[2] This finding also substantiates the Mind-body Connection. Not only do our thoughts and emotions affect our physical body, activity of the body stimulates our brain!

---

2 *Los Angeles Times*, Health Section, Feb. 10, 2003

IMPORTANCE OF THE LYMPH SYSTEM

The lymph system, a series of tubular ducts and nodes throughout the body is designed to clean out and eliminate Cancer cells, as well as bacteria, viruses and other harmful molecules. It is your body's garbage disposal system. This system has no pump as the arterial system does in the heart, and is a one-way- only transit of lymph fluid through the ducts to the lymph-nodes, sponge-like tear-drop shape organisms that act as filters. Valves are used to keep the lymph fluid from flowing backwards

Since there is no pump for lymph fluid, a thin, watery liquid, as there is the heart for the blood, the one and only and best way to activate its healing and cleansing power is to initiate exercise that employs muscular contraction. During exercise, the rate of lymph flow can increase from three to fourteen times its resting rate, carrying out wastes and Cancer cells much faster.

In other words, your lymph system is your clean-out system. Removing lymph nodes to diagnose and "stage" Cancer is one of the Medical Establishment's worst mistakes, as they cannot be put back into the body. A major impairment of the immune and healing system thus results. It's like taking out your garbage disposal system to see if there is any waste-matter in it, and then throwing it out even if it is clean!

This removal can also lead to a serious disease called Lymphedema that can cause swelling and paralysis, infection and even death. The lymph fluid travels with its Cancer cells to the sponge-like nodes to filter and clean out these cells. If the nodes are surgically removed, the lymph fluid is stuck, which is what causes the inflammation and paralysis. It has been blocked from doing its job.

My Mother's friend, Eda, had her lymph nodes removed when she had surgery for Breast Cancer. Toward the end of her life, the Lymphedema became so bad, causing her arm to became so grossly enlarged and paralyzed that she could not even dress herself!

For Lymphedema, massaging the valves of the lymph ducts can help. Gravity can also help pull the fluid through as in rebounding or jumping rope. This helps recycle the lymph fluid that will stagnate when a person is confined to bed or has a sedentary lifestyle, causing toxins to accumulate resulting in fatigue as the body slows in ridding itself of infection, bacteria, viruses, and Cancer cells.

Judy Taylor is considered one of the foremost Lymphologists in the U.S. She has designed Lymphatic Certification classes for Medical Doctors, Registered Nurses, Acupuncturists and Naturopathic Doctors. She has also designed, in conjunction with an Engineer, a Lympholine, a re-bounder built to become the missing lymphatic pump supporting detoxification. Instead of a rigid frame and steel post legs, the Lympholine has a full suspension system like a car. The whole rebounder, including the legs, moves with you every time you jump on it. This allows you to float as you head skyward.

Fortunately for me, Judy lives in Los Angeles. I called to interview her and she graciously invited me to her beautiful West-side apartment where she helps people with various disorders by supporting the lymph system with her Lympholine, massage, and Gua sha. This is an Oriental practice of a scraping movement of the skin first applied with oils and then rubbed with a jade burnishing tool that helps draw out stagnant intercellular fluids to the surface from deep within

the body. Dry brushing with a large bristle brush is also recommended to stimulate lymph circulation.

I came to her apartment with my own batch of trauma.
The Cable Company had backed into my studio building
breaking my wall into two horizontal parts and putting out
the electricity for my saw. I am also an artist who paints
large-scale paintings. This is where my canvases are built
and stretched and a stack of new ones would be completely
endangered by rain coming into my building via the hole in
my wall! I had spent a frazzled day interviewing contrac-
tors, calling my attorney, and fighting with the Insurance
Adjuster while worrying about the consequences if I didn't
win my battles. To say I was stressed out would put it very
mildly. I was a nervous wreck!

I asked Judy if I could try her Lympholine. She led me
immediately to her patio where this handsome black, high-
tech mini-trampoline awaited me. I stepped on and began to
jump and float heavenward. Instantaneously, I was light and
free and full of joy, as happy as a child dancing and jumping!
Tensions flowed out of me so readily it was as if I could watch
them vacate my premises! It felt so good to be rid of the fear
and distress the damage to my studio had left on my own
interior environment. I was suddenly giddy with happiness,
laughing, and carefree as a lark! My body did feel cleaner as
I stepped down. Cleansed, refreshed, and released as if from
a prison of grief, worry, and tension.

Judy, a beautiful woman in mid-life, is also a Cancer
survivor. In 1978 she was diagnosed with thyroid Cancer.
She submitted to surgery to remove her thyroid and also her

tonsils. The lymph-system, composed of lymphatic vessels and lymph nodes, works in conjunction with the bone marrow, appendix, spleen, thymus, and tonsils to keep the body clean. Thus removing lymph nodes and tonsils cripples the immune system. The tonsils I had removed when I was six perhaps contributed to my first Cancer scare, the lump in my neck.

After the operation, Judy was then was put in a lead-lined room and given an iron cup of radiation to drink! Everyone else ran hastily out of the room! Incredibly, twenty-five years later, she still has a high level of radiation in her body from this so-called treatment!

I asked her how she manages not to have a recurrence of Cancer.

"I work at it!" she exclaimed. She became a Lymphologist, turning her obstacle of having had Cancer into an opportunity to help others learn how to heal. This is a Principal of healing—turning obstacles into a path to help others. In the next Chapter, the lymph system will be closely linked to how you live your life. But to close this chapter on exercise, the key to getting well from Cancer lies in energetic aerobic exercise alternating with rest. Every study supports the fact that exercise works to prevent and heal Cancer. Drinking plenty of water throughout the day will also help clean and refresh the body's cells.

By getting into a regular exercise routine everyday, your body will be pointed into the direction of full, beautiful, energetic and robust health. It's only a matter of time until you are well again!

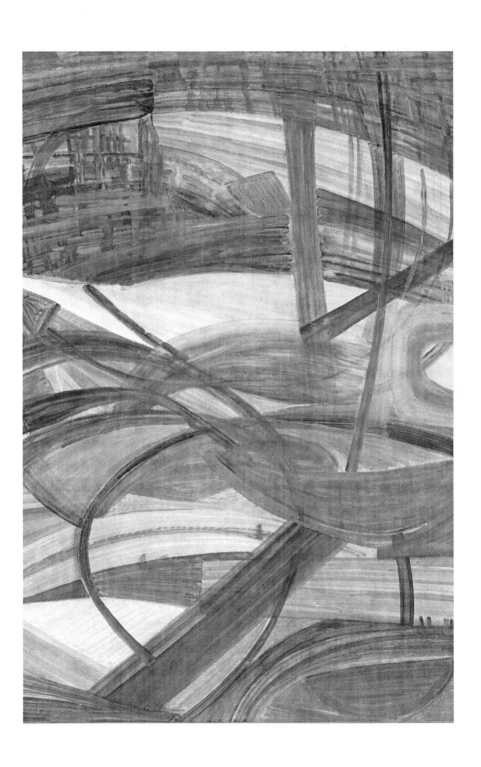

CHAPTER 10

Some Profound Thoughts on Getting Well from Cancer from Lymphatic Expert Judy Taylor

ORIGINALLY I WENT over to Judy Taylor's lovely apartment to learn more about the Lymph System for my exercise chapter. But as she spoke, I realized that she was going to be much more profound and deep about the subject of Cancer. After seeing Cancer patients for many years, she had much more crucial information to convey. Following is my interview with her.

Q. "Judy, what exactly is the lymph system?"

A. "The Lymph system is the garbage disposal system of the body, but it is also the mirror reflection of how we live our lives," she began, startling me with this spiritual approach to a subject I thought was only mechanical.

Q. "You mean the lymph ducts and glands are not just a mechanical cleansing system?"

A. "Absolutely not. Lymph works with the emotions, with what we eat, and how we communicate or repress communication. Lymph is the flow of life, and like the flow of the ocean it needs to keep moving in order to detoxify the cells. It cleanses and washes cells. Lymph holds memory; the cells hold memory, so when we hold onto anger or repress other feelings and words, when we are tense, tight, and stiff, this creates stress which in turn causes blockages of energy, flow, and blocks in all aspects of our life.

Q. "How does exercise contribute to lymph system function?"

A. "Exercise absorbs trauma. The lymph system is three times larger than the blood system and in order to keep it moving *we* have to move. If we become sluggish, the lymph fluid thickens and can become stagnant. This builds toxins because the lymph can't move them to the nodes that act as filters. Infections can occur from these toxins and become a disease."

Q. "How exactly does releasing stress help?"

A. "In releasing stress with exercise, you are saving your life. Holding onto stress is toxic to the body. We have to honor ourselves and let go of judgment and blame. *Healing has to do with believing*. We have to know that life is giving us circumstances for a reason."

"Yes," I agreed. "My building's wall is torn apart, yet I feel lucky."

Judy looked startled.

"I am lucky because the building is old and rebuilding that wall is probably just what it needs. It is, in all probability, decayed, eaten away by termites, water-damaged, and consumed by dry rot," I laughed. "It probably gave way quite easily like a piece of old cardboard! Now the Insurance Company will rebuild it for me with new, strong wood and plaster!"

"Yes," Judy agreed. "You can see the glass is half empty. Or you can see the glass is half full. It's your call. It's your pick and choice."

Q. "Do you think nutrition has a role in Cancer?"

A. "Of course," Judy acknowledged. Stress has to do with thoughts and beliefs. But also you can stress your immune system with certain foods such as sugar, too much salt, caffeine, alcohol, carbonated drinks, over-charred barbecue, dairy foods, hormones and antibiotics given to animals and eaten as meat. Eating non-organic food that is sprayed with chemicals can stress the system as can medicines and drugs."

Q. "But psychological factors also come into play?"

A. "Definitely. Repressed communication is conflict. We don't love ourselves enough to express who we really are. We use blame, shame, and judgment. We haven't any right, really, to judge ourselves or others. I found in breast issues, in Breast Cancer, the lack of ability to stand for who we really are, grief, sadness, lack of nurturing, and lack of self-love are the big initiators."

Q. "What else helps the lymph system to conquer Cancer?"

A. "Yoga is very good. And deep breathing, meditating and learning to release deep stress. Getting in touch with who we are with clarity. We need balance in all areas of our life. We especially need to let go of trauma, emotional and parent issues that distress us.

Q. "Do you have any examples to relate?"

A. "I had a beautiful, wealthy patient. She had everything. She was gorgeous and had all the money she could ever need to find help to get well. She had Breast Cancer and got rid of it. She traveled the world working with many kinds of healers. She ate very well and exercised.

Then she got it again. Once more she healed. The third time she got Breast Cancer she died at age fifty. She never could let go of the anger she felt about her mother. Even after her mother was dead, she still could not forgive her for past hurts and the way she was treated. Although she learned how to heal from Cancer, I believe that the anger that she could never release finally killed her. I absolutely believe if she could have found the strength to forgive her mother for past injustices, for whatever she perceived as hurtful treatment or wrongful punishment, she would still be alive today."

Q. "She could not release anger from the past. That is what killed her?"

A. "We have to live in the moment. We must let go of the past, otherwise we have no future. Living in the past, we miss out on everything. Look at what this woman lost—maybe fifty more years of life—mostly because she could not forgive her mother."

Q. "How else does stress adversely affect your health, and how does exercise alleviate it?"

A. "When you are stressed, your breath often becomes shallow. Exercise forces you to breathe. You must oxygenate your cells to keep them healthy."

Q. "What else can we do to have healthy cells?"

A. "Find ways to have fun! Life gets heavy and hard. Watch children. They move around all the time. They laugh. If they fall down and cry, they get up again. The next minute they are laughing again. It's all over and done. Learn the process of letting go."

Q. "Anything else?"

A. "Watch your weight. Obesity is toxic since fat cells collect pesticides and chemicals where it stores them. Eat good fats such as Omega three fats—fish oil, flax, olive oil, nuts and cold-water fish.

Overeating saturated fats in meat and dairy products reduces the immune system's ability to flow, overtaxes it. Cancer cells can thrive when the immune system is overloaded and clogged up with fat and toxins."

Q. "What is the most important thing to do to get well from Cancer?"

A. "There isn't one thing. It's important to do a whole program."

Q. "But isn't there a crucial first step, the will to live?"

A. "Yes. I do think there is one crucial decision one must make first if faced with a diagnosis of Cancer. *That is you must make the decision that you want to get well.* You must desire to get well. You must sincerely want to turn your health around and be willing to do the necessary work. You must take responsibility for your health. You must take responsibility to change your life"

Q. "Is it ever too late?"

A. "You can get well at the ninth hour. I've seen people who were so sick they couldn't walk. They come to me and get well. If you can get sick, then you can get well."

Q. "What message would you like to impart to people with Cancer?"

A. "Tell people that information is power. We must educate wisely for ourselves. Don't hand it over to others to do it for you. Find out everything you can by reading, looking at the Internet, asking questions, going to the Medical Library and reading Alternative health books. Make your own decisions. Empower yourself."

I thanked Judy profusely. She had given me so much more wisdom than I had sought. I gave her a warm hug and a copy of my revised Breast Cancer book. As I drove home, I felt I had learned some more deep lessons about Cancer, its causes, its prevention, and its path of healing.

CHAPTER 11

The Healing Power of Love

I BEGAN AN e-mail correspondence at the end of 2002 with Shin-ichiro Terayama, a Japanese Cancer survivor who healed himself after medical treatment failure using the power of love. Here is our correspondence:

Dec. 30, 2002

Dear Susan,

I cannot see your face and hear your voice, but I am able to feel your vibration in Japan.

Thank you so much for your e- mail so I could know more about you. I shall try to find your book on Amazon.com.

I understand your effort to change the Conventional Medical world. Where are you living now?

Dear Shin,

I live in Los Angeles. Years ago, I healed myself of Breast and Uterine Cancer step-by-step on an all-natural health program. I heard you used natural means to finally get well, mainly love.

Dear Susan,

I was an executive director of the Japanese Holistic Society, established in 1987, for eight years. While I was in a process of my healing Cancer, step-by-step as you did, I met some Medical doctors who were trying to study holistic medicine. We started in 1987.

They tried to understand my requirements by using their mental, cognitive abilities, using educational abilities, but they could not feel the true meaning of holistic medicine that I wanted to convey to them.

So finally I said to them if they try to conceptualize it, they won't succeed. The true way to study holistic medicine is to suffer from Cancer and heal it. But they didn't get it. All the doctors who suffered from Cancer died!

They tried to be very scientific and applied many methods they believed were holistic but they used them in a non-holistic way. It was not deep but very shallow.

This is my introduction and short message. I am sixty-seven years old and very healthy. I am a Physicist and am still working as a scientist. I travel to many countries and give talks and workshops.

Susan: Why didn't those doctors understand your message?

Shin: Healing takes creativity and imagination. It is an art! That is why you as an Artist understood creative healing, whereas those Doctors who wanted to be Scientific didn't get it and died!

Susan: You have to believe in what the Buddhists call the Mystic Law of Cause and Effect and be able to implement this law.

Shin: It takes an extraordinary person to have the character to not go with the conformity that Cancer treatment presents.

Susan: You are an extraordinary person! I found you on the Internet and I found a treasure! I am fifty-eight and very healthy and youthful. I am alive because I learned about health the hard way. I took responsibility for my own path to wellness.

Shin: You have to learn to love your disease! Now about one-third of the people in Japan die of Cancer and this statistic is increasing year by year. I was a Cancer patient near death in the hospital in 1985. I returned home and healed myself through natural healing. Loving your disease, using games, meditation, sharing, and praying. All these lead to a spiritual awakening. For the participants who are able to open their heart, they can get the true wisdom of healing.

Susan: Where did you find this out?

Shin: Findhorn, in the Northern part of Scotland by the North Sea. I had Cancer in my right lung. Creativity helped me find a path to healing. I love music. I was helped by playing my

Cello. Music is healing. Findhorn, like Esalen, is a loving, healing environment. For forty days, I concentrated on love. I loved my Cancer and hugged everyone. It was forty days filled with absolute, pure love.

On returning to Japan, I went to a hospital to have an X-Ray exam and my Lung Cancer could not be found. It had disappeared.

Susan: What happened, exactly, in Findhorn? How did you get the Cancer to go away?

Shin: At Findhorn, they do a lot of "body work." This may help people open their Chakras. Everyone is treated as a real human being. Conventional Medicine might consider transforming its healing capabilities by introducing a more humane attitude toward people seeking Medical help.

Susan: So you go around the world to try to explain how to heal from Cancer naturally with the power of love?

Shin: Thirteen years ago, I was invited by Findhorn to speak and then afterwards I went to India twice. India is very dear to me. It is a wonderful, deep country. I think in my former life I lived in India! I talk about learning to love, sending love to your tumor or Cancer, thus healing it.

Susan: Did you detoxify your body?

Shin: Fasting is the most powerful detoxification of all. Proper juicing and whole grains are important for healing. In Cancer you need nutrition. You have to restore vitamins lost in stress.

Susan: Tell me more about your healing journey.

Shin: At first, my Cancer was in my right kidney and I was treated by conventional medicine: surgery, chemotherapy, and radiation.

Then while I was being treated in the hospital, staying there for five months, my Cancer metastasized to my right lung and rectum.

Susan: Often a major stress, a distress, precedes the Cancer by eighteen months to two years or more. Did you have a major stress in your life?

Shin: The first Kidney Cancer came from emotion when I was threatened by one of my clients. I believe it is true that Cancer comes from negative emotions.

Susan: How did you find the courage to check yourself out of the hospital and embark on your own natural healing journey?

Shin: During my stay at the hospital for five months, I felt tremendous pain from the treatment of my Cancer by Chemotherapy. In addition, I was getting weaker after thirty treatments of high-energy radiation.

I saw many people die by the main effect (I don't think it is a side-effect) of Chemotherapy and radiation while I was in the hospital. I just wanted to escape from that routine treatment.

I feel war is not the answer. Waging war on this disease does not get lasting results.

I sent deep love to my Cancer that I created by myself. At bedtime, I would practice getting into a state of profound love and send this to my tumor.

One night I had a very strange dream that I was watching my body from above. It was a scene from my funeral. I wanted so badly to return to my body! I shouted that I still wanted to be alive and present in my living body!

I didn't believe an ordinary scientist like me could put any credence in dreams like this at the time. Now I feel it was some kind of near-death experience. After this dream, my sense of smell increased strongly and I could not stay in the bedroom of the hospital especially at night when the door was closed.

One night I left my room and finally found the place on the rooftop of the hospital where there was no smell. I stayed there all night. My doctor was very upset because he was very afraid of suicide, jumping off that roof! He came to the hospital early that morning and asked me if I intended to return to my home. I said, "Yes."

I did not obey the doctor's orders to get checked every month. Instead I went in every six months. It was my intuition, beyond my scientific training as a physicist, that I didn't need all those check-ups.

I founded the Japanese Holistic Medical Society while I still had a tumor because I had a strong belief that my Cancer was being reversed by intuitive healing.

Susan: What did these doctors think?

Shin: I tried to re-educate these Medical doctors, but they had no sensitivity and were very stubborn. After eight years, I left the society that I founded with the Medical doctors. In 1988, I was invited to the Findhorn Foundation a speaker on the future of politics in the spiritual world. I connected with a Jewish-American woman staying at the holistic retreat. She had stayed at Findhorn for two years. It is a wonderful, spiritual healing place.

I got really interested in spiritual healing, intuitive healing, healing with the power of love. I visited Esalen in March 1989 and attended the American Holistic Medical Association conference in Seattle, Washington. After that I revisited Esalen five times and Findhorn nineteen times.

At an alternative medicine conference, I met Andrew Weil who invited me to visit his home in Tucson in 1990. I subsequently have visited him ten times and lectured to his students about increasing high sensitivity of the human power to heal. In turn I invited Andrew to Japan, coordinating his lectures and workshops. This month I am leaving for India. We can discuss healing in more depth when I return.

Love, Shin

LOVE VERSUS REJECTION

O. Carl Simonton who invented visualization talks about Cancer beginning in childhood with parents not accepting their child as he or she is. He points to the first seeds of Cancer originating in "basic rejection." When we don't get the love we need as children due to our parents having their own conflicts and turmoil and being physically, spiritually, and emotionally unable to give it, the cells are deprived of this basic nurturing. Later on in life, in times of distress, this lack may cause our cells to run amok.

For Shin, it started with a threat from his client. Or perhaps it actually started as an infant when his mother was unable to give him the love he needed because she was not receiving the love she needed from his father. Deprived of this, he had to learn to love himself.

Shin talks about being in a loving, accepting environment. He sought this out instinctively knowing that in order to get well, he needed this type of cocoon to wrap himself in. His stressed and deprived cells needed the physical warmth, acceptance, hugs, and putting himself in a loving place.

Human warmth and human touch have proved over and over again to be an important healing ingredient in disease.

Even in animals this turns out to be true. Confoundedly, rabbits fed a high fat diet compared to rabbits fed a low-fat diet were actually healthier. Upon further investigation, the rabbits with the miserable diet were the ones the caretakers picked up and hugged when they cleaned their cages at night after the scientific investigators went home!

Breast Cancer patients often have trouble dealing with relationship conflicts with their mothers. Sending love to our mothers, whether they are still alive or not, can help us in our own healing capacities. Whether or not she had the interest or ability to love us is not as important as the love we can give back to her. She gave us life. We have the ability to acknowledge this with our love.

If anger and resentment, jealousy and fear are the negative emotions, which pave the way to illness, then love can shine a path back to health. Shin proved it. Lung and Brain Cancers cannot be cured by the Medical Establishments "routine" treatments. However, Shin overcame one of the most difficult forms of carcinoma, Lung Cancer, by using his power to love.

Who can you forgive and love today?

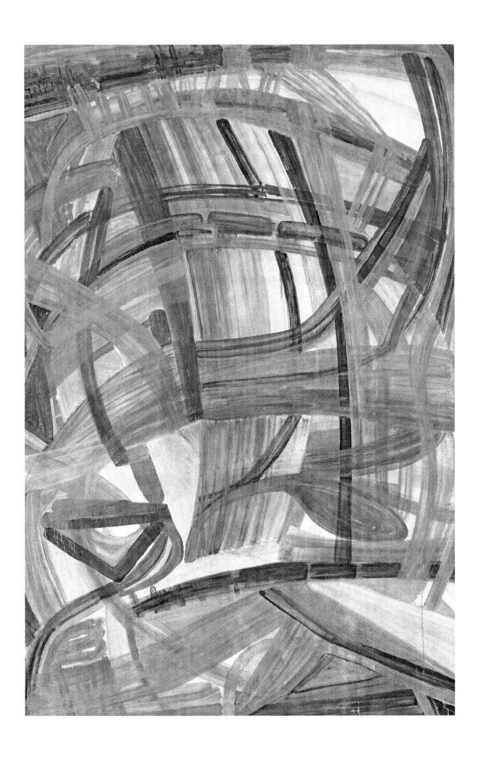

CHAPTER 12

"Saying Everything but Good-Bye"
Creating Spiritual Healing Energy

WHEN SHE WAS really sick with Cervical Cancer, Rosemary Fairchild began a second career—resurrecting her singing voice, recording a CD, "Forever American," and traveling the world giving concerts. One of her songs seems especially apropos: "Saying Everything but Good-bye."

I visited Rosemary in Whittier, California in the house she grew up in that she has totally cleaned out and redecorated in a light, airy, contemporary way. A large picture window overlooked the whole Valley below, green with rows of Cyprus trees and flowers. "This is my favorite time of day," she told me joyfully, as the sun began to sink, shedding a luminous red-orange glow onto the endless sky. Surprisingly, although I came to her tree-shaded contemporary home to talk about her suffering from Cancer, I feel enveloped in a deep sense of peace, security, and beauty.

She practices Buddhism, chanting Nam-Myoho-Renge-Kyo to a Gohonzon, a scroll with calligraphy enshrined within a wooden cabinet called a Butsadon. She chants at least one hour a day. "I'm a leader," she told me proudly. I practice too and have watched Rosemary's phenomenal growth as a human being over the years despite her Cancer.

"It was work or die," she told me frankly. "You need the confidence that you can awaken the power within your life-force that can cure any illness! You need to suspend disbelief and trust the mystic law. You can overcome any obstacle with prayer."

"Do you credit prayer for extending your life over the medical treatment you received?" I asked her.

"The AMA is a wicked piece of business!" she laughs. "I fired my Oncologist. Get your radiation from the sun and your platinum (Cisplatin, the Chemotherapy), from the jewelry store! You need the stand-alone spirit. You can get well, but you have to make the effort yourself."

Rosemary had been through enough suffering for her fifty years to enable her to be an expert on the subject. She had weathered thirty-one operations and was contemplating her thirty-second on her foot.

When her Cervical Cancer was diagnosed, she had a radical hysterectomy. Her bladder was so full of Cancer they did another operation to cut out major parts of it and rebuild it. They put tubes in her kidney. She also subjected herself to a lot of radiation, having treatments every day from October to February using high dose beams. After twelve hours of Chemotherapy, which she calls, "The Devil's Dildo," she stopped these sessions. She submitted to "Dr. Burn, Dr. Poison, and Dr. Butcher" because she "had so much Cancer." She felt capable of dying in a moment and, she admits, it actually became an "attractive option." When she asked the radiologist how others got through so much treatment, he told her that no one else had lived to complete that much radiation!

She experienced severe problems with her nervous system from these radiation treatments.

She also fell some months later and injured her leg. A metal rod was surgically inserted which led to problems in her foot. Subsequently, she cannot walk easily or stand for hours on the stage to perform her concerts. She also developed infections in her face and eye and had another metal plate inserted into her cheek.

The more Rosemary talked about her Cancer, multiple surgeries, radiation, Chemotherapy, and the consequences of these dangerous treatments, the more in awe of her I became. I began to seriously take note of her appearance and what she was doing as she spoke to me. Overweight when I met her some years ago, she now was seriously obese, at least one hundred or more pounds overweight. As Rosemary talked, she reached for her cigarettes, which I objected to, so she opened a bottle of Scotch instead. "I like whiskey too," she joked. Later she rolled a joint!

How is this lady alive and talking to me? I wondered. She knew about my book and my MOTEP program, but she hadn't read it. I made sure to give her a copy before I left. But I wondered if my advice would be futile. She admitted she could not exercise due to her health problems. Truly, the one and only thing that was saving this lady was her strong spirit, as she didn't seem to have any health habits! That is why she is good for this chapter on the spiritual aspect of getting well. Rosemary's spirit was the one and only thing keeping this lady alive!

"Read the April 6 Daily Guidance," she advised me. Later at home I opened the book, confirming her advice on how to chant without a feeling of pain and sorrow:

"If your heart is controlled by your complaints and dissatisfaction, the Buddhist gods will not activate, and you will be unable to accumulate good fortune toward your enlightenment.

"On the other hand, if you have a strong sense of appreciation and joy deep within, you will see fortune and benefits shine even more brightly in your life and receive increased protection from the Buddhist gods. This is the essential truth of faith."

I also looked at the preceding guidance while I was at it:

"The purpose of faith is to attain enlightenment, which means absolute happiness. We began our practice to become happy, but why do we have to meet with so many obstacles? It is because we need these trials called obstacles to mold a diamond-like, indestructible 'self' of Budhahood within us."

Although I am a tried and true advocate of the MOTEP program, that is looking scrupulously after your health and eliminating health-destructive habits that Rosemary paraded in front of me, I realized that the health factor that possibly matters most is happiness, joy, and a spiritual commitment. To practice some sort of prayer every day, morning and evening, whatever your faith, might protect your life more than even giving up self- destructive habits will. Of course, I still advise creating health in all ways possible. Rosemary's attitude is really remarkable as she lives with constant pain from **all** her treatments and operations, as well as her illnesses and accidents. She can no longer stand on the stage to give her concerts. Yet she does not let any of it get her down! And because she is so limited, Rosemary is creating a musical instead! When this production is finished, she expects to be well enough to be able to stand and participate in it.

She advises, "Stay out of the hospital. Use reason and confidence." She emphasizes that in Buddhism, chanting brings "actual proof." And she points out that Buddhism is "win or lose."

"You can win in your daily life," she laughs. "You have to mutate or die!"

"I see you won," I remarked gleefully. "You have over-come tremendous difficulties and pain,"

"You have the power to transform anything," she pointed out. "The mind is the only thing in the way."

"Did you have a big stress two years or so before you got Cancer?"

"Yes, I lost friends and relatives, twenty-five people I cared about. Maybe I wasn't aware of my depression. Twelve of my friends died from AIDS including my little brother who was only thirty-four. My grandparents, uncles and friends all passed away. I had a close girl friend that died at age forty for no apparent reason. She was not overweight, had no bad habits. She spent Saturday night with her niece, as she was single after two divorces. They would make dinner together and then watch TV. She was lying on the couch enjoying some show and she died! I never figured it out, and no one else did either. She had a lot of friends, a good job, and was always funny and sweet.

"The world is full of distress. The thing is not to be swayed by events. Focus on what you can do. I built a second career as a singer. During the first career, I developed a benign tumor that wrapped around my vocal chords! This took several operations. So when I took up singing again, I had to rebuild my voice first!"

"How did you get so much courage to go through all this and still create this stunning record album?" I asked, amazed. "How did this lovely music come out of your Cancer?"

"People are afraid. But you have the power to awaken in your life the ability to cure any illness. Refuse to hand your power over to anyone else, whether it is a Medical Institution, Doctor, Alternative practitioner or Guru. Refuse to be limited. I had no interest in succumbing to fears. I knew I could get well. I knew I could do it myself."

"Did you have any special reason to reclaim your health?"

"Yes, my parents lost one child. I am determined to outlive my parents and not make them go through another great loss. My mother is eighty-eight and is slowly losing her health now. She was never one to be sick."

"How important is the spiritual aspect in getting well?"

"I wouldn't have made it without it. It gave me confidence and I knew from past experiences that I could show *actual proof*. I knew I could transform anything."

"You are living proof!" I complimented her.

We traded her CD for my book on Breast Cancer and we hugged. I left the beautiful area not only with songs to play later, but a song in my heart.

SELF-DESTRUCTIVE HABITS CAN DESTROY YOU

In stark contrast to Rosemary, Kari gave up her self-destructive habits and now lives without pain in a most vibrant and happy mode. She also now looks like a model for *Shape* magazine. I asked Kari to write about her spiritual journey on her road to wellness. This is what she wrote five months into her self-healing:

"My spiritual healing began five years ago when I got clean and sober. At the time I was spiritually bankrupt and so had to start at zero.

"The first thing I had to do was to ask for help from others. I was not in a position to help anyone else. Everyday I had to make a gratitude list and pray, thanking my higher power for all my good fortune.

"This is the most healing attitude, an attitude of gratitude. Going around bemoaning my misfortune would have sent me in the opposite direction from what I wanted. Now I can actually help others, which is one of my spiritual exercises. Whether it is giving someone a ride, helping the elderly, helping someone move, or anything similar. I consider it to be an essential part of my spiritual program.

"Another important activity is connecting with Nature. Making an effort to get away from the stress of the city can bring instant healing to any difficult situation I might be carrying on my back. I find this connection to be very important in modern times.

"Then I have to pray for others, especially people I resent or have feelings of hostility toward. That may be the hardest part of my spiritual program. It is not just to help them.

Mostly, I admit, it is to help myself because resentment is poison to the body.

"Also I have to make the effort to smile from my heart many times a day and laugh to release pressure. Sometimes looking at a situation with humor is the most healing thing to do. I'm working on finding a way to laugh at/with Cancer.

"Spirituality to me is also practicing random acts of kindness to strangers when there is nothing in it for me. For example, in traffic, to let someone in, instead of rushing ahead and cursing at the same time. The best kind of act of kindness is the type when the receiving power knows nothing about it, let alone who or where it came from. Those are, of course, the hardest for me and therefore the most powerful. When it's just between me and my higher power, not trying to take credit, or tooting my own horn, so to speak—this is the most spiritual and the most healing good turn."

Both Rosemary and Kari have found that the spiritual path is the high road to healing Cancer. However, if both women were standing side by side, the contrast would be stunning. While neither of these women looks ill and both are in great spirits, Kari has a youthful body that she shaped up with her exercise program and took care of with her nutritional menu and juicing. She looked and felt terrific. Her opting to give up drugs, alcohol, smoking and the constant search for escape from reality by using these substances abusively, led to a vibrant, lifestyle free from pain and complaints. She is joyful with her new discoveries and almost totally healed.

On the other hand, Rosemary has not opted to give up self-destructive habits, looked older than her age, and is full of pain, disability, and physical complaints. Spirituality, to me, includes nurturing the body. Just as the mind cannot really be separated from the body when it comes to our health, the body's health will, in turn, influence our thoughts and feelings. It is a two-way deal.

To get well from Cancer, I found that taking rigorous care of myself, physically, mentally, and spiritually, and giving up self-destructive habits such as overeating, were essential building blocks to restoring my full health. Prayer and chanting were most important to heal the mental components of the disease. Still the two tumors I had were physical proof that my body needed to be taken care of. Along with establishing peace within my mind, I did the hard work of physical healing and regeneration.

In *The Buddhist Path to Simplicity*, Christina Feldman writes, "Each time we get lost in our obsessions and cravings, we deprive ourselves of the simplicity, contentment, and freedom that is to be found in a single moment embraced with intention and the willingness to be touched by its richness. An ancient Sufi saying tells us, "Within your own house lies the treasure of joy, so why do you go begging from door to door?"

THE HEALING SPIRIT

The very first step in spiritual healing is to establish a feeling of peace within yourself through spiritual practices. The body cannot do the work of healing when the spirit is depressed, angry, frustrated, jealous, resentful, and/or feels the need for revenge. Forgiving those who have hurt us and asking forgiveness for those we have hurt, even if the request is not met with appreciation, is the first step to self-healing

Cancer. We cannot be responsible for those who will not forgive us for past behavior they judged as unacceptable, even when we whole-heartedly apologize. However, we can make the effort to apologize, and this, in itself, is a healing tool.

In Buddhism, we chant for their happiness. We also do this for those who have caused us pain. At first this was the hardest concept of Buddhism for me to accept. Why should someone's happiness, a person who hurt me, be prayed for? But I did it anyway, if grudgingly, and I found, to my sheer amazement, that it worked! Not every time, of course, or right away. Sometimes people are slow to forgive or to "come around." Patience with people, compassion, and of utmost importance, letting go of your own hostile feelings, often will turn a bad situation around. Above all, appreciation for what they *have* given you, both telling them and including it in your prayers also helps. Being at war with others is being at war with yourself. Cancer cells are at war with the normal cells. To heal Cancer, proclaim a truce!

When praying or chanting for yourself and others, visualize the ultimate results you want to achieve. Picture yourself happy, healthy and successful, living the life you always wanted, a life filled with joy and love. Visualize a friendly meeting between you and someone you view as an enemy or have a turbulent relationship with. Form a picture of yourself back to full health, smiling and laughing, singing, traveling, dancing, creating art, playing music, writing, loving, and enjoying a full, rich wonderful life.

Your endorphins, hormones of happiness and healing, will flow, your immune system will fill with white blood cells, and your Cancer won't have a chance, under these spiritual conditions, to continue to grow. Cancer cells will be blocked by your strong "Will to Live," and your spiritual practice. Soon they will disappear on their own.

Both Rosemary, who according to the Doctors should be terminal by now, and Kari who took charge of her body, mind, and spirit instead of handing her Breast Cancer over to the Medical establishment for mutilation and poisoning and might, by now, be fighting recurrences and side-effects, have defied their prognosis. They have chosen the spiritual path to staying alive!

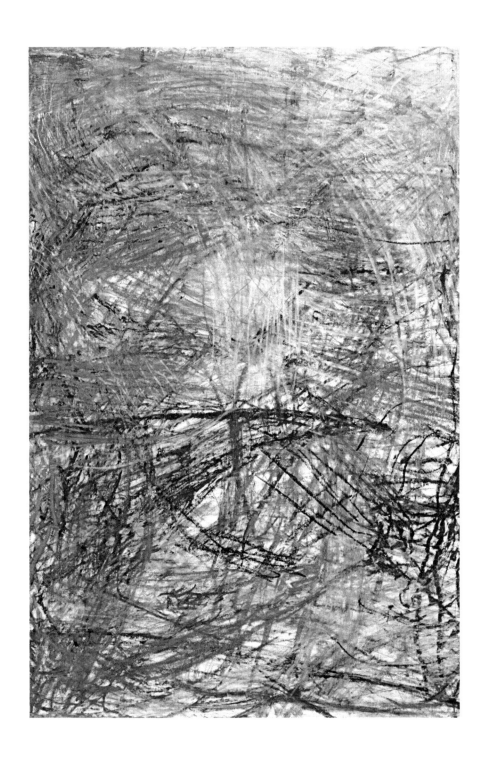

CHAPTER 13

The Emotional Core of Cancer

CANCER IS AN emotional disease.

You may have not read this statement before. Your doctor has not, in all probability, mentioned it. In fact your doctor probably has not asked you any questions such as are you happy? Or how is your love life? Doctors are trained in diagnosis. After they figure out through a surgical biopsy that you have Cancer, they are trained to offer "treatments." These basically consist of surgery, chemotherapy and radiation. If they are truthful, they will tell you that you have a fifty percent chance of living five years more or less with these treatments, depending on your stage of Cancer. They may even give you a tragic prognosis of a few months.

Doctors don't ask the personal questions that would help you understand why you have Cancer or go through any understanding of the core of the disease and its healing, which is the emotions. *Without changing the core of how you store your painful emotions and allow them to destroy your body, any treatment is only temporary.* The Cancer may, sooner or later, recur.

LORRAINE'S BATTLE

Lorraine, age forty-three, was diagnosed with Cervical Cancer in 1994. The stage, after two biopsies, was diagnosed as micro-invasive. The treatment recommended was a hysterectomy, which would mean she could not have a child. She refused treatment, as she wanted children. She left the doctor and focused on her version of treatment: deep meditation. This seemed to do the trick. She had a son.

When Lorraine wanted a second child, a few years later, her husband was opposed to the idea. She got pregnant anyway. The second child wouldn't come out and had to be cut out with a Caesarian section. Lorraine was also diagnosed with Ovarian Cancer. Again she chose as her treatment deep meditation. She also submitted to a hysterectomy, by then content with having the children she wanted.

In 1997 Lorraine again had pain and was once more diagnosed with Cancer in the same area. The treatment was "low dose" radiation, although the technician misread the treatment and gave her a high six-thousand Rad dose, twice as much as he was supposed to aim at her. Lorraine was told she also needed Chemotherapy or she would die. She refused and focused on self-healing.

Lorraine and her husband fell on hard times in the year 2000. Her husband lost his job and subsequently, in six months, they were thrown out of their house. They lived with friends or on the street. Their son began a downhill course of drugs, theft and intermittent stays at Juvenile Hall.

Lorraine was deeply upset. For no apparent reason, she began to throw up once a month. She would feel perfectly fine and suddenly become nauseous and vomit. At that point, there was no money or insurance to go to the doctor. Her husband, an artist who does murals and film work, finally found mural work. They found another home and reestablished themselves.

However, that December, she was diagnosed with Grade Three Endometrial Cancer, the lining of the uterus. No surgery was recommended, as there was too much scar tissue. She had had a "horrible" biopsy with six-inch long needles and what looked like a cake-icing tube that acted like a gun. She got a huge inflammation from this Stereotactic biopsy. By then, she was through with Medical diagnosis and treatments and didn't stay for their recommendations. She walked out of the door.

That was when I met her.

She read my book on self-healing of Breast and Uterine Cancer, began to see Dr. James Privitera who gave her enzymes. She tried to schedule a time to come to see me to talk about her situation. But every time she was planning to come to my studio, she had to cancel. Her son was in trouble, her husband was an alcoholic, she felt unwell—she related one trauma after another. Her life was one of extreme distress, pain, illness, complaints, and severe problems.

Lorraine finally arrived one Friday morning. She was a beautiful woman of about the right weight. She didn't look a bit ill. I congratulated her on getting this far, defying all Medical prognoses. And then I explained how she stuffed her painful emotions in the same spot, her lower torso. Her life, full of frustration and pain, was being cut short because she let these painful emotions eat away at her, always in the same area of her body.

Lorraine explained she was also an artist. She had dreams of doing an "Earth" project. She could visualize what she wanted to create. However, she had pushed this project aside, thinking that her husband was the artist in the family, while she played the role of wife and mother.

I pointed out her blocked creativity and how she allowed painful emotions to destroy her will to live, stuffing them into her lower torso, her creative center.

"You have had the same pattern for forty years of your life," I said. "You have learned to do the same thing with your frustrations and anger, direct them into your lower torso," I explained.

I recommended she do three things to change the pattern she had subconsciously fallen into. She wrote these down to practice at home:

1. Acknowledge your painful emotion: fear, doubt, anger, frustration, jealousy, or feelings of wanting revenge.

2. Put the situation that created these feelings "out there." "You're in here, while the situation is over there. Do not put this problem into your body," I explained.

3. Do something positive with the energy created by this emotion. For instance, take out some paper and watercolors and start sketching your "Earth" project you dreamed about.

I stood up and twirled around and around. "You do this," I said. "You go around and around and the results are always the same: Cancer in the same area. This is where you put your negative emotions. That is where the problems show up."

"Give yourself credit," I told her. "You defied the odds. You had two children you were told you could not have. You survived diagnosis of Cervical, Ovarian, and Endometrial Cancer. And you laugh because at one visit, Doctors weren't sure exactly which Cancer it was! Yet here you are, a beautiful woman, alive and talking to me."

Tears came into her eyes. "I'm afraid to be myself!" she admitted.

"You have fallen into a pattern and you can change that pattern," I encouraged her. "You just have to recognize it and do those three things".

I explained to her the tremendous stresses I had been under. My studio was now repaired in the nick of time. The rain my contractor and I had worked so hard to beat, repairing the hole in my wall caused by someone backing their truck into my studio, had fallen in torrents the very night after the workman had removed their tools and wheelbarrows. We had tremendous rains that would have ruined my studio, my paintings, and my storage of books.

Now the neighbor and I had to argue and fight about rebuilding the block wall for their parking lot that was built too close to my wall, a mere three inches, blocking the water which then leaked into my studio, causing severe water damage to my property and to my paintings.

I hadn't been able to show my work to collectors while the studio was being repaired and was not compensated for this by the insurance company. My galleries were not selling either. Once again I was struggling financially.

"Yet I have had several people lately tell me how good I look! Several people said I 'glowed' and asked me if I had either gained or lost weight! Maybe I had lost a couple of pounds, but basically, my weight is stable and has been since high school.

"How healthy you are is not dependent on external circumstances, but how you internalize those stresses." I explained to her. "As an example, I had one relative who survived the worst Concentration Camp, Bergen-Belson, where Anne Frank and my Grandparents died of starvation and illness. He was the only one of my family to survive, even though they knocked out all his teeth. He eventually came to America where I met him. At that point he was well over eighty years old, but nevertheless the best-looking, most handsome and elegant man in the hotel room at my cousin's wedding! He had lived a life of a rascal and scoundrel. He had cleverly lived off women all his life. I think he had a lot of fun. Nothing got to him. He never had to work a day of his life in order to enjoy his upscale lifestyle!

"How did he survive one of the worst concentration camps? He must have used his wits and beauty to scheme and talk his way into survival against all odds. When Typhoid swept the camp putting the final nail in the coffin of my starving grandparents, he survived and healed.

"I danced with this wonderful, clever, and gorgeous man. My cousin, the survivor!"

Lorraine and I did a white-light meditation together. We visualized a white, laser-like light streaming from our eyes or third-eye in the middle of our forehead. We then took it through our bodies—neck, breasts, arms, stomach, lower torso, thighs, knees, lower legs, and feet. We used this light to cleanse, remove tension, and feel very relaxed, as the white light is a spiritual light. "Accept it as your healing source," I advised. We did this for twenty minutes.

"That felt really good!" Lorraine said. She hugged me. She left with her "homework," a new way to deal with her negative emotions and an exercise to clean her body of tensions and Cancer-causing blocks. She also had an "assignment" to get back in tune with her creativity by going back to doing her art. She badly needed to remove that block. Lorraine left with a clearer vision of why and how she developed Cancer and a new pathway to healing and total health.

THE TYPE C PERSONALITY

Anger is the major emotion in Cancer—that is buried and unacknowledged anger. The "Type C" personality as described in Lydia Temoshok's insightful book, *The Type C Personality*, is the "too nice" people-pleaser, intent on being accepted and acceptable at all costs. Under this guise of pleasant and cheerful personality lies buried anger. And while love is fearless, anger is fearful. Covering our anger with a pleasant façade of what we believe is presentable and conforming behavior, breeds a strong resentment. This buried anger and resentment will eventually turn into negative energy that destroys our very cells.

According to the book, *The Heart of the Soul*, by Gary Zukov and Linda Francis, anger is the agony of believing that you are not capable of being understood, and that you are not being understood. Beneath anger lies pain, and beneath pain lies fear. Burying this anger, I believe, creates disease.

An individual who is continually angry is in continual pain, according to Zukov and Francis. **Buried anger and pain can kill you.**

Also, Zukov and Francis write, the core cause of anger is lack of self-worth. Buried anger, covered over with a façade of pleasantness, then must be a form of acting. If this description fits many Cancer patients, then their hold on reality is, perhaps, tenuous. Hiding their feelings because they do not want to upset anyone pays off badly in illness. Anger is energy that has to go somewhere. If it is buried, the body may create a tumor to protect itself from destroyed cells, cells that have been mutated from strong hormones caused by anger that is not acknowledged or released in creative, physical, or emotional activity.

There are constructive ways to express or deal with anger. One does not have to start screaming. Taking positive action, going for a walk, exercising at the gym, talking to friends about the problems, or just beating a pillow, helps to release these tensions.

Confronting people who have hurt or insulted us takes tremendous courage for many of us, especially those raised in authoritarian, punitive households. One's self-esteem is often tested by others, especially if they are insecure. This ability to stand up to them can be cultivated a bit at a time. Practice communicating your feelings. Be willing to apologize, also, for hurting or insulting others. This is also important as a healing gesture. However, many Cancer patients have played the doormat role for too much of their life. People have walked over them or used them as scapegoats. They have not found the strength to stand up and insist on better treatment for themselves.

Women, especially, are vulnerable to criticism and abuse. We often take on the subservient role that damages our self-esteem. Standing up for yourself takes practice, courage, and self-respect. These can be developed with practice. The rewards are great. You will become a stronger, healthier person for not becoming intimidated by others, for standing your ground.

Cancer can be a very intimidating diagnosis. Stand up to it! Be determined to beat it and heal. **Mental and spiritual strength are the most important components in your healing program**. Cancer responds to mental suggestion. You have the power to visualize yourself well!

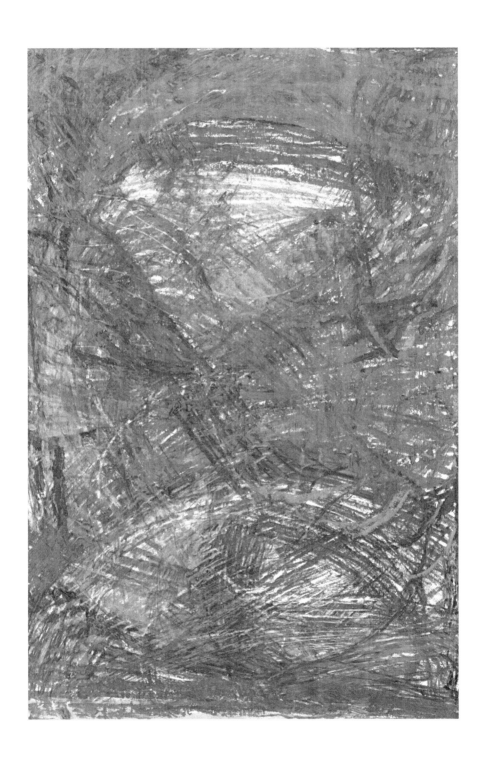

CHAPTER 14

A Healing Sisterhood—Brandon Bays' Incredible Shrinking Tumor

A SISTERHOOD OF Healing now exists. Many women have healed themselves of tumors and Cancer. Not only have they been able to live to tell about it, they went still further to write books, record audio and video tapes, speak to large audiences, and even develop new careers helping others to learn natural approaches to getting well from Cancer.

Eydie Mae Hundsberger, perhaps, began the trend many years ago when she wrote, *Eydie Mae, How I Conquered Breast Cancer Naturally*. This remarkable woman decided to switch her diet to all natural raw foods, mainly vegetables and fruits to reverse her Cancer. She may have based her ideas on two former leaders in Nutrition for Cancer: Max Gerson and Ann Wigmore. She found her body's ability to heal itself when she went on this vitamin and enzyme-enriched diet.

Dr. Max Gerson was a pioneering doctor who would take Cancer patients in, at times on stretchers, after treatment failure. They came to him devastated by the so-called treatments called "conventional" and "standard" today. He would give them fresh squeezed vegetable juices throughout the day as their "routine" treatment. When they could eat again, he gave them only organic, primarily vegetarian food. This detoxification process resulted in many "cures" for these "incurables."

But rather than use the word "cure," a misleading word to me, I would describe this as unloading the body of toxins, waste products stuck in the colon, and excess stress hormones, allowing the body to *heal* itself. As you can readily see, there is a vast difference in a "cure" that is some miraculous substance we might or might not find and that is outside ourselves, and healing that involves an interior process of getting well utilizing the body's own resources, repair mechanisms, and wisdom.

Gerson describes fifty cases that miraculously went from terminally ill patients to vibrant living humans in his book, *A Cancer Therapy: Results of Fifty Cases and the Cure of Advanced Cancer by Diet Therapy: A Summary of Thirty Years of Clinical Experimentation.* His patients went through a total healing, so other complaints such as allergies disappeared. Charlotte Gerson, his daughter, carries on the tradition at the Gerson clinic in Mexico. Here we have the word "cure" to mean inner healing and with complete inner healing comes little or no threat of recurrence.

Ann Wigmore, another pioneer, wrote the book, *Be Your Own Doctor,* in which she describes taking Cancer patients in at her Hippocrates Institute, exercising them, and giving them fresh wheat-grass juice to drink along with a diet of organic food, mostly fruit and vegetables. Her book is an inspiration and foundation for body regeneration.

Ann Frahm found herself dying from the Medical Treatment of Cancer before she decided to quit that route and go on a self-healing path using Nutrition. In her book, *A Cancer Battle Plan*, Ann describes the grueling, destructive Chemotherapy and radiation she underwent, as well as the high-dose Chemotherapy used in the Autologous stem-cell "transplant," where stem-cells are removed from the body and stored in a freezer while the body is inundated with toxic drugs. The stem cells are then reinserted to "rescue" the patient. The idea of bringing the patient close to death, and then rescuing them was, at best, inane. This horrendous Frankenstein- Meets-Cinderella like fairy-tale invention has been mainly discontinued as it was found to mostly kill off or terribly disable the immune system as well as almost destroy the gastrointestinal tract of the patients who submitted to it. Many of them died soon after this procedure. Without an immune system, they were totally vulnerable and might succumb to even the smallest infection, as my young friend Kimberly did.

When I met Ann, she was gorgeous and healthy. She was using her experience to speak to the large group of people who gather at Lorraine Rosenthal's Cancer Control Convention every year. She was a quiet, introverted person who had obviously found out how to get well the hard way. But, unfortunately, nutrition is only one aspect of Cancer healing. Either because she did not address the psychological problems that she also needed to work on, or her immune system was too jeopardized and compromised by her Medical Treatment, she died of a recurrence some years after I met her. Still she lived a healthy life for many years after she was given a terminal prognosis.

The Psychological side of Cancer healing, which I believe is crucial to address, was written about by self-healer, Alice

Hopper Epstein, in her book, *Mind, Fantasy, and Healing— One Woman's Journey from Conflict and Illness to Wholeness and Health.* In it, she describes going on an interior probing of her psyche in order to unearth what was disturbing her and the various fantasy scenarios she conjured up to relax her mind into a state where healing could take place. Alice does not speak of changing her diet, juicing, exercise, or prayer. While changing only one aspect of life after discovering a problem area *can* produce complete healing, MOTEP emphasizes the importance of a complete life-changing program, including healing distress and grief along with the detoxification diet and exercise. Yet she was able to create a peaceful state of mind wherein the body could accomplish its self-healing task without changing any other physical aspects of her life.

BRANDON BAYS' HEALING CAMPFIRE

Two inspirational and important books emphasize changing one's life and focusing on a healing journey after a diagnosis of a tumor or Cancer. Brandon Bays, *The Journey— A Practical Guide to Healing Your Life and Setting Yourself Free,* will be discussed in this chapter. In the next chapter, we will look at Cheryl Canfield's journey to wellness and a new life free of Cancer.

Brandon Bays calls Cancer a "gift" and a "wake-up" call. She was called upon to tap her inner healing resources when, despite leading a healthy lifestyle, she developed Cancer. Some of her health practices included being a vegetarian, drinking filtered water, and even doing re-bounding on her mini-trampoline every day in Malibu, California where she breathed clean, fresh air, living with a loving husband and children. Despite all this, she was diagnosed with a basket-ball-sized stomach tumor!

How could this happen to a woman with healthy habits who had spent her career as a therapist? She wondered to no avail at first why a woman who had traveled the world giving health seminars and learning everything she could about how the body heals itself could develop such a gigantic tumor. It had grown from her pubic area all the way up to her rib cage! The doctor told her in no uncertain terms that surgery was her *only* option. Pushing her, as many doctors do when they discover a tumor, she was told the surgery would have to be done immediately!

Brandon told the doctor that she was a mind-body healer and asked how much time could she have? But the doctor was adamant about surgery because Brandon was experiencing bleeding and might die within the next few days. Her mass was also "too big" to consider alternative healing, the doctor pointed out. Gesturing to a shelf full of books, the doctor said, "There is not one case history in all these books of a woman who has healed naturally from a pelvic mass the size of yours." After a half an hour of horrendous negotiation and wrangling, the doctor finally agreed to "give" Brandon one month to try to heal herself!

Brandon knew she could heal the tumor; the only question was not *if* but how.

As in my own healing experience, Brandon first of all took responsibility. She knew she was responsible for creating the tumor and she would also be responsible for getting rid of it. Secondly, she began her journey by cutting out all caffeine from her diet. Caffeine destroys the self-repair mechanism of the cells according to research done at Occidental College.

Thirdly, Brandon decided to trust her body in the self-healing process. Everything happens for a reason and purpose, she acknowledged. She decided she would finally have to get in touch and release negative emotional issues stored in her cells. She also began a fresh vegetable juicing program and regular massage to get the lymphatic system flowing.

Still she felt the most important aspect of her healing journey was to get to the core of the tumor that she felt was *emotional*. This took courage and patience. The emotional memories stored in the cells must be dealt with. She prayed, with all her heart, to be finally able to face them. Brandon felt she had stayed in denial a very long time, repressing the pain. Expanding into stillness was her way to dive into this previously prohibited area. As she dove into the tumor using an inward journey, Brandon found fear and an old childhood trauma she thought she had finished with. She found other emotional disturbances too that she had masked by putting on a brave face.

She imagined a campfire and put all the people in her memory around it. The younger version of herself began to talk to them. Her parents were there and explained their behavior by recounting how her little sister had drowned at age four.

Still she had to dig deeper. Finally she heard the voice during one of her meditations, a nameless voice telling her, "You have to forgive your parents."

Brandon reconstructed the campfire, putting her parents around it. The younger version of herself then forgave her parents in the innocent way children forgive. She began to cry. She knew the story was over.

The next day on the massage table she began to feel a subtle but palpable energy coursing through her arms and legs. As she left the table she felt woozy and wobbly. Reaching for her stomach, she found the tumor had softened. She went home to rest in bed.

In the morning she felt the molecules of her body buzzing and shifting, just as I had experienced in my breast on my own healing journey. It had felt like bees inside my breast as the white blood cells and cytokines were breaking down my rock-solid tumor. The next three days she was weak and disoriented as her body went around going about what it knows instinctively how to do. The wisdom of the body, just as mine had, took over the healing. Brandon felt that rather than the tumor clinging to her, she had clung to the tumor as it protected her from her hurtful memories. In that way the tumor had been useful to her. *When Brandon acknowledged the pain she had gotten from her family and forgave them, she no longer had any functional use for the tumor.*

Two days before her Doctor's appointment, she continually felt her stomach and realized that, although she still had some of the tumor, it had gone down in size very dramatically.

During her Doctor's appointment, she remembered that a year earlier a pap smear had come up pre-Cancerous. The Doctor noted a big improvement in the tumor. She acknowledged it had gone down in size from a basketball to the size of a six-inch cantaloupe melon! "That's a significant change," the doctor told her. "But it's not significant enough. You still need it surgically removed."

The doctor was impressed, but told Brandon that the tumor was volatile and could blow up again.

"You need to get real about this, Brandon," she said. "This is not something to be taken lightly."

Even though everything the doctor said made sense to her, Brandon still found herself saying "NO!" She told the doctor that she didn't believe the tumor would blow up again. She was on a healing journey and would continue that journey without the "help" of a surgeon, thank you very much!

Brandon decided not to travel anywhere, even as she had an opportunity just then. She decided to give herself completely over to her healing journey. She had made so much progress and was very encouraged despite the doctor's extreme pessimism. Her friend Skipper suggested she leave her doctor and go to a large hospital with high-tech equipment for tests in two more weeks. Encouraged, she gave herself that deadline. Over the next week-and-a-half the tumor continued to shrink.

It was during that time her massage therapist said, "Brandon—I just have the feeling that there is nothing there. I can't feel it with my hands no matter how deeply I dig."

At the hospital two weeks later, Brandon felt excited and scared. She was taken to an Ultrasound machine that would enable the doctor to see her organs clearly. Brandon decided not to tell her whole story to the doctor but to get her fresh unbiased opinion. She just told her she was thirty-nine years old and her gynecologist felt she needed a thorough exam. She might have a small growth in her uterus.

The doctor then wanted a comprehensive exam. After she turned off the monitor, she said in a delighted tone, "Well, first off I'm not finding anything." She turned to more high-tech machinery to make sure. She found nothing in the uterus and her ovaries were clean. Finally she exclaimed, "You're textbook perfect clean!"

In six-and-a-half weeks she had completely dissolved a basketball-sized tumor. (I had gotten rid of both breast and uterine tumors in almost the same amount of time—one week short of two months or seven weeks.)

TRUST THE INTELLIGENCE OF THE BODY

Brandon admits she didn't do all the work. She says, "In fact, I didn't even heal myself—the infinite intelligence inside did all the healing". It was a journey of discovery for her involving surrendering and letting go. *Brandon felt the most important point was forgiving all the people involved in her pain and letting go of all the stored anger and resentment.*

She then felt the tumor was a *gift*. That it had formed for a reason and that reason was to teach her how to heal and help others to learn this urgent lesson. No one else can do it for them, she realized. It had to be a journey of discovery unique to each person.

The pattern of the cells had to be changed and needed be renewed with healthier cells. (The liver cells take six weeks to regenerate, the skin cells only three- to-four and you get a new stomach lining in four days. The eye cells completely replicate every two days.)

Yet you must change the pattern, otherwise the same

disease process will show up in the next generation of cells. That pattern of how the cells relate often holds "phantom memories" according to Deepak Chopra, who Brandon went to hear speak. Healing must take place at the cellular level.

She realized to really help people, she must get them to realize that there is no need to turn to anyone or anything outside of themselves.

I, too, often tell people who are diagnosed with Cancer, "You don't have to go anywhere. *Your body will heal itself wherever you are.*"

Brandon has used her healing journey to help others. She offers campfire seminars. Participants put the people who matter to them around it and go through emotional layers to find what they are troubled by, the emotional cause of their physical maladies, whatever they may be. She has them forgive, completely and utterly, the participants of past injuries to their soul and spirit. Often their "presence" issues a wake-up call. People suddenly realize that the anger they hold against others is what is destroying their health.

Brandon Bays goes around the world teaching people about emotional healing to get their health back. Her book is a bestseller. Anyone interested can read her book or enroll in her Healing Journey seminars. Her journey of self-awareness and healing has helped thousands of people. She is a great example for us all.

BRANDON'S STEPS TO HEAL CANCER

Let us review the steps she took in her healing journey that were similar to mine:

1. She took total responsibility for her health.

2. She set a deadline, negotiated with her Doctor, as I did with my Doctor.

3. She worked hard to meet that deadline in several ways. She went on a juicing-detoxification program as well as began her emotional detective work, going on an intense inner journey. She prayed sincerely and with all her heart to find her emotional blocks and anger. When Brandon found she held on to resentment towards her parents, she visualized putting them around a campfire and forgave them with all her heart.

4. She let go, surrendered, and let her body do its innate healing supported by her message therapist, her juicing program, her prayers, and her emotional work and forgiveness program.

5. She trusted her body completely to do the work while supporting it in every way possible. Brandon absolutely *believed* she could do a self-lumpectomy, even though her tumor was huge, a veritable basketball in her pelvis and stomach.

6. When she saw progress, reducing her basketball to a cantaloupe, even though she did not completely meet her first deadline, she refused to think negatively— give in to surgery— but set a second deadline.

7. After her miraculous victory and all-clear report, Brandon set about using her methods of healing tumors and Cancer to help others, sharing her crucial information in workshops and lectures as well as writing a book.

My hat is off to Brandon Bays. She discovered exactly the same thing I discovered. The body will heal itself of Cancer and Tumors without Medical Treatment when supported in every way by a sincere whole body-mind healing program. This program supports the body's own innate healing ability instead of mutilating and poisoning it with Medical Treatments. With enough encouragement, will power, and a plan to reclaim your health, self-healing will begin to take place. Spontaneous remission is hard work. It isn't all magic. But the body has the miracle ingredients to make tumors and Cancer disappear. There definitely is a mystical element that defies scientific explanations. It involves trusting the healing wisdom of the body and supporting its healing abilities in every way you possibly can.

CHAPTER 15

Cheryl Canfield's Profound Healing

AFTER A HEATED, emotionally charged argument with her second husband, Cheryl Canfield experienced sharp pains in her abdomen. The pain was so sharp that it brought her to her knees. She was tired of fighting with him and had, in fact, been tired for months.

Going to the Doctor, Cheryl was devastated to find herself diagnosed with advanced Cervical Cancer. A lump was also found in her breast, and although it was biopsied as benign, the Cervical Cancer was found to be invasive. The diagnosis "didn't seem possible." She felt she wasn't a candidate for Cancer. She practiced Hatha yoga daily, ate a balanced vegetarian diet, and meditated. On top of that she led a retreat center and taught others steps toward inner peace! She felt humiliated.

Was she a hypocrite to teach others how to live a healthy life when she had invasive Cancer?

A complicated surgery was recommended as the *only* route for her to follow, a Medical route that was so extreme that after the Surgical Oncologist described it, with its devastation and mutilation to her body, Cheryl was sure she would die on the operating table.

She said "no" to the radical surgery to her Doctor's astonishment. Cheryl told her Doctor that she would rather face death on her own terms. "I'm not afraid to die," she told her doctor and went off to do just that.

Cheryl's Doctor wrote a letter to her describing a terrible, wasting and rotting death that was certainly in no way preferable to extreme surgery that would have her coping with her waste products with catheters and bags. He begged her to reconsider submitting to the radical surgery.

She realized her core problem: her body was overloaded with years of emotional stress and loss.

Without the surgery, she knew she might die, but she also knew it wasn't inevitable. "No one can predict death," she writes. Cheryl opted to trust her intuition. She decided to begin her research. This led her to move out of the house she shared with a man she couldn't resolve problems with, rent an apartment, and go on what began as facing death but instead turned into her very own personal healing journey. Her book, *Profound Healing: The Power of Acceptance on the Path to Wellness* relates her path back to health.

STARTING THE JOURNEY

Cheryl began by going to Mexico. There she found Alternative Clinics that offered combinations of Laetrile, chelation, nutrition, live cell therapy and other alternatives. Although she didn't feel drawn to any particular program, she did stock up on several months' supply of Laetrile, and a six –month supply of herbal tonic, calcium, iron pills, Pau D'Arco tea, and enzymes.

Since none of the clinics interested her, Cheryl decided she had to start working out her own plan.

At first she decided she was "exploring death." She was terrified of the miserable rotting death her doctor had described, so much so that she began to do some research on how to take her own life!

Thankfully, that idea abated when Cheryl realized her life plan was not to be cut short. It just wasn't her time to take leave of this earth she called home. With her little dog Plato, she began a simple life in a tiny apartment, giving up the usual tempo and productivity she was used to. She devoted herself only to her own care, preparing juices and taking vitamins, laughing that her kitchen looked like a pharmacy.

She recognized her tiredness and began sleeping at various times throughout the day. "Sleep became my other world," she writes. Cheryl began to pay attention to her dreams. In one of her dreams, she met with a group of people who would do projects involving the manipulation of energy. One of the dreamed projects was manipulating the energy of the earth along its fault lines. At other times the meeting dissolved into a prayer meeting in a circle of light. At these times, her body felt extremely light, composed more of energy than matter.

In other dreams, she was alone with a teacher. The teacher told her she wasn't absorbing B vitamins very efficiently and she should give more attention to balancing her diet.

She had the most active sleep-state, as her subconscious imparted information to her about the next steps in her healing process. Cheryl was open to listening to her dreams and began to start a journal to record them and to write about other insights as to what she should do to heal.

She began to give up the idea that she was going to die. "Nature has always been a model for me," she writes. "I trusted my body's natural process." She felt that if her body was producing a profusion of Cancer cells, there must be a reason. "Find out everything you can about Cancer and then follow your intuition," she decided.

OXYGEN WIPES OUT CANCER

Further research revealed that Cancer doesn't grow in oxygen. Cheryl put this research into practical use and took up jogging. At first Cheryl was so weak that she could barely jog half a block. Slowly, however, she built up her endurance. Over her year's healing journey, she managed to slowly build up to three miles! This made her proud and she felt stronger.

In her little new community, she found a population of homeless people. She began to seek out these people with her friendship. They loved her dog Plato and looked forward to seeing the two of them jogging or walking around town. She helped one Cancer victim, Bob, by suggesting he stop drinking and smoking and reconcile with his daughter he was estranged from. Bob began to resolve his feelings of powerlessness in dealing with the events of his life. In turn, I believe she received the healing energy one gets when one reaches out to help others.

Cheryl's research revealed the prevailing attitude about Cancer, how attempts to control and overpower the condition resulted in overkill and destroying healthy cells like the inevitable civilian casualties in a war.

She disagreed with the battleground concept. Simply cutting out Cancer cells was ignoring an important message. "What was Cancer telling me?" she wondered.

She decided to visualize her Cancer cells as young, unreasoning children. Bombarded by years of stress, they felt their lives were threatened. She embraced her Cancer cells, assuring them that they were no longer alone or helpless. They could stop reproducing. "I was in charge now," she decided.

She felt an instant response of peacefulness throughout her body. A profound healing experience was taking place.

DEAPENING A SENSE OF APPRECIATION

She began to start each day with a deep sense of appreciation and gratitude for the day ahead of her and to scan the inside of her body to see what she could find. Often she would feel good, but sometimes she felt jabbing pains in her lower abdomen. If that happened she would rest her hands, palms down, on her stomach and feel the radiant energy being released to the painful area.

In every situation, Cheryl believed she could find opportunities to grow, to learn, and to teach, to give and to receive. She realized that she had held onto resentment towards many people in her life. She began to write letters to these people in her journal and make up letters that they would write back to her. She began to comprehend that forgiveness was really about taking responsibility for herself and resentment only held her in bondage to that person. This is a profound lesson she discovered and led her to write a series of forgiveness letters. (In this way each person could go their own way without the blocking from strings of resentment).

"If we're willing to look deep enough, I discovered, we can see that no good comes from making another person the bad guy; blaming others only keeps us stuck in the role of victim."

She began to see that the key to her exercises in forgiveness was honesty. "To really heal, I knew I had to be completely honest with myself and find a way over each hump, one at a time.

" One of the most difficult challenges was coming to terms with the loss of a relationship, (her first marriage), that I had thought would be lifelong."

This was so tough that she cried, agonized and even yearned to be someone else.

Eventually, she got to the other side. Cheryl decided to like herself as she recounted her good and bad qualities and decided she had enough of the good!

She encountered years of built up resentment and anger toward her ex-husband who had left her. She wrote a letter pouring out her pain to him in her journal. She realized that "my wholeness and happiness come from within, not from circumstances or people outside of me. I live with a basic joyfulness about life simply because I choose to."

When she needed financial assistance from her year off work, she applied for government assistance and was persistent until she got her checks.

THE OPPORTUNITY TO DO HEALING WORK

Although this healing journey took a year and was a lot of hard, intensive work, she writes,

"I appreciated the opportunity to be doing this work. It had come as a result of dealing with Cancer, which I was also coming to appreciate in itself. Teachers come in many forms."

She set a goal or deadline to be able to witness the birth of her first grandchild.

At the end of the year, Cheryl made the decision to go back to her original doctor for another pap smear. The results came back normal—class 1. She felt it was a miracle!

The Doctor wasn't satisfied and wanted to do another colposcopy, to see what was happening at a deeper level. She stayed for that test too.

After waiting weeks, Cheryl finally was informed that all her cells were normal. But, the doctor told her, "The tests didn't mean anything."

Doubts crept into her mind and she began to feel pains in her abdomen again.

But then she forgot the doctors and the tests when her new grandson, Nathaniel, was born. She began to feel good, took long walks, and found she had more energy during the day. She decided to go to another doctor.

The new doctor commended her for the strength of her convictions. She noted that the tissues she was taking a pap smear of looked pink and healthy and noted what good shape Cheryl was in. When the tests came back normal, the doctor told her that her tests certainly weren't meaningless. "If it doesn't show Cancer, you don't have Cancer."

"Do you think you are in remission?" her daughter asked her hopefully.

"Oh, no," Cheryl replied, laughing. "Remission sounds like there's something hanging over my shoulder waiting to pounce. I don't know what's going to happen tomorrow or next year. I only know that today I am well."

So Cheryl Canfield ends her description of self-lumpectomy and her healing of invasive Cervical Cancer that was "supposed" to kill her She took total responsibility for her health, refusing complicated surgery that she felt would destroy her.

CHERYL'S MIRACLE OF SELF-HEALING

1. She took total responsibility for her health, refusing a complicated surgery that she felt would destroy her. *She realized that disease cannot be cut out of the body.*

2. She was willing to do the research to find out what would work best for her own healing program. She researched the Mexican clinics, bought some of their products, but decided that getting well was a do-it-yourself project.

3. Cheryl set a deadline when her daughter got pregnant as to be able to see the birth of her new grandchild.

4. She let go of an emotionally disturbing relationship and moved to a small apartment with her dog Plato to either die peacefully or to get well.

5. Cheryl began to believe that she could get well.

6. Appreciation for her life and gratitude for each new day found its way into her consciousness. *She found the will to live.*

7. Cheryl found a way to help others, discovering relationships with homeless people could actually bring her inner peace and healing energy.

8. Journal writing became important to her as a form of self-discovery, expressing forgiveness while letting go of resentment that tied her to people in a negative way.

9. Her research uncovered the important fact that Cancer cells cannot live and grow in an oxygenated environment. She began a mini-jogging program, slowly and surely building up to a three-mile run.

10. She found a method of visualization that would work for her, visualizing embracing her Cancer cells as frightened, runaway children and giving them the love and security they so badly needed.

11. When Cheryl ran out of money she applied for government assistance and was persistent until she got it.

12. She discovered it was not enough to kill or get rid of Cancer cells. She learned that Cancer was a lesson. *Cheryl was privileged to have Cancer so she could find out what this severe teacher was trying to impart to her.*

13. Her lessons seem to be the following: love yourself, let go of resentment by forgiving others, take laetrile and vitamins and eat balanced vegetarian meals to rebuild strength, establish a feeling of peace within yourself to create a healing environment. Do your own research into what Cancer is all about, the latest findings, how others healed, but use your own intuition to make decisions, set a deadline using an important event, take up an exercise plan to create an oxygenated internal environment. Helping others is an important aspect of healing. Get lots of rest and sleep and pay attention to your dreams. Be patient with your body, as it took time to get sick and it will take many months to get well. When you feel you are well, go back to the doctors who won't believe you are healed even when the tests prove you are normal once again!

Once more, we are privileged to read of a healing journey that took courage, strength, and fortitude. Validating the time-tested truism of the body's capability to heal itself of disease, even life-threatening invasive Cancer, Cheryl Canfield wrote her heroic story. What is yours?

CHAPTER 16

Healing with Faith

DON WENT OFF to college, following his own direction calling himself the "classic prodigal son." But he found he didn't like the academic environment. He became unhappy and dissatisfied with his life on his own.

Eventually, he decided to return home. To fit in, Don cut his hair and shaved his beard. When he did this, he found a fairly large, unsightly mole on his face. He went to the doctor to have it removed and thought everything would be fine once it was gone.

However, several days later the physician called and asked Don to come back to see him. He said that the mole indicated he might have Cancer and that he should consult some specialists. Don went to see an Oncologist. The Cancer doctor said Don had Lymphatic Cancer, which had metastasized throughout his body. They needed to schedule immediate radical surgery in order to remove it.

"I asked them what would happen if I underwent this surgery, and they basically told me that they gave me a sixty percent chance to live," Don said.

At that point he asked them what would happen if he didn't have the surgery.

"Well, you may live six months at the most," was the pessimistic reply.

Don felt very frightened by this. But, interestingly enough, he began to recall being raised in a Christian Science oriented home, where his family relied on God for healing and guidance. At age seven, he had been healed of an earache by studying the Christian Science Bible Lesson, outlined in the *Christian Science Quarterly.*

THE POWER OF PRAYER

This and other healings reminded Don that it was time to turn to God. Although Don's past healings were microscopic compared to his present problem—invasive, metastasized Lymphoma, they were proof to him of God's goodness and power. "This reassurance enabled me to handle the initial fear that I was going to die and gave me some kind of hope," he says. "I realized that these doctors were very conscientious and were following their highest sense of right. But they really didn't have a cure for this disease. They couldn't really tell me what had caused it or anything much about it, except that it could kill me."

Don made his decision. He would turn whole-heartedly to God and rely on prayer for healing.

He contacted a former Sunday school teacher who was also a Christian Science practitioner and asked her to pray for him. She had him read Mary Baker Eddy's *Science and Health* and contact the practitioner each day.

Some days Don read one page and at other times he read a whole chapter. He would call her to discuss what he had read and report his progress each day. He read that the cause of all sickness was "fear, ignorance, or sin." He began to comprehend that negative states of thought, mentally entertained, were being manifested outwardly in the form of illness.

"My initial reason for reading *Science and Health* was to be healed, but I found after a while that I was becoming more interested in simply knowing God. In fact I almost forgot about my original reason for doing this reading."

After three months, he felt completely healed. He underwent several rigorous physical examinations by doctors, and there was no trace of illness. This happened twenty years ago and he still passes his physicals with no problems showing up![1]

HEALING WITH FAITH

Don dealt with his disease by finding hope and using the power of faith to self-heal.

In my own case, I found that chanting and following Buddhist concepts helped in healing my Breast and Uterine Cancer. Many Buddhists have healed themselves of life-threatening Cancer when they chanted Nam-Myho-Renge-Kyo to a Gohonzon, or shrine. We decorate this shrine with fruit and living plants, candles and incense, and have a gong, which we strike before and during our ceremony. Each of us has a shrine in our own home, and we also gather for group chants. Buddhism teaches about Karma, the simultaneity of cause and effect. This teaches us to take full responsibility for everything that happens in our lives.

THE POWER OF FAITH CAN HEAL SUFFERINGS

President Ikeda writes, *"It is the power of your faith that can change the sufferings of body and mind into*

---

1 *Christian Science Sentinel* Special Report

true happiness. How deep your faith in the Gohonzon is, how strong and pure it is, or how patiently you persist in your practice—these determine everything in your future."

In Buddhism, you chant and pray, expecting to get what you are chanting for. That is, you are not "hoping" to get well. You set a deadline, and *expect* to meet that deadline. This works amazingly well for other goals too. Of course you "make causes" to reach your goals. You take action!

Praying and chanting work on the subconscious level. Recognizing a higher power brings a mystical support system to your aid. It brings peace into your soul, enabling your immune and healing systems to function at their peak. Chanting and praying can elevate your life condition, too

THE TEN WORLDS

In Buddhism there are ten worlds. These are ten states or conditions of life that we experience within ourselves. They are then manifested throughout all aspects of our lives. Each moment we can go up and down in these worlds. Here are the six lower worlds:

Hell—This is a state of suffering and despair, in which we perceive we have no freedom of action. It is characterized by the impulse to destroy ourselves and everything around us.

Hunger—Hunger is the state of being controlled by insatiable desire for money, power, status, or whatever. While desires are inherent in any of the Ten Worlds, in this state we are at the mercy of our cravings and cannot control them.

Animality—In this state, we are ruled by instinct. We exhibit neither reason nor moral sense nor the ability to make long-range judgments. In the world of Animality, we operate by the law of the jungle. We will not hesitate to take advantage of those weaker than ourselves and fawn on those who are stronger.

Anger—In this state, awareness of ego emerges, it is a selfish, greedy, distorted ego, determined to best others at all costs and seeing everything as a potential threat to itself. In this state we value only ourselves and tend to hold others in contempt. We are strongly attached to the idea of our own superiority and cannot bear to admit that anyone exceeds us in anything.

Humanity (also called Tranquility)—This is a flat, passive state of life, from which we can easily shift into the lower four worlds. While we may generally behave in a humane fashion in this state, we are highly vulnerable to strong external influences.

Heaven (or Rapture)—This is a state of intense joy stemming, for example, from the fulfillment of some desire, a sense of physical well-being or inner contentment. Though intense, the joy experienced in this state is short-lived and also vulnerable to external influences.

THE HIGHER STATES OF CONSCIOUSNESS

Learning—In this state we seek the truth through the teachings or experience of others.

Realization—This State is similar to Learning except we seek the truth not through other's teachings, but through our own direct perception of the world.

Learning and Realization are together called the "two vehicles." Realizing the impermanence of things, people in these states have won a measure of independence and are no longer prisoner to their own reactions. However, there is great potential for egotism in these paths, and contempt for others who are not on this level.

In the course of a day, we experience different states from moment to moment in response to our interaction with the environment. For instance, the viewing of another's suffering might call forth the compassionate world of Bodhisatva. Bodhisatvas are those who aspire to achieve enlightenment and at the same time are equally determined to enable all other beings to do the same. We devote ourselves to alleviating others' suffering. There is great satisfaction to be found in altruistic behavior.

The loss of a loved one might plunge us into Hell.

However, these states will not control us, nor will we define ourselves in terms of them when we achieve the highest state. Our nine worlds will be harmonized and function to benefit both ourselves and those around us.

WE ARE ONE WITH OUR ENVIRONMENT

In Buddhism we are not separate from the environment. Rather, the environment is a reflection, a mirror of ourselves. The effects of karma (our own actions) appear in the environment. Whichever of the ten worlds an individual manifests will be reflected in the environment. For instance, a person in the world of Animality will perceive the environment as a jungle where only the strong survive.

BUDDHISM AND CANCER

Considering all this, how does Buddhism affect Cancer? Chanting and reviewing my own karma helped me to heal in the following ways. I began to take a hard look at my life to see the problem areas:

1. Buddhism teaches you to take responsibility for whatever happens to you.

2. Chanting itself creates healing power. Nam Myoho Renge Kyo roughly translates to: "The mystic law of cause and effect through sound vibration. Chanting is like the "roar of the lion." What disease can therefore exist?

3. Buddhism helped me to review the "causes" of my illness. How did my body deteriorate into disease? I suffered financial setbacks from a recession where people stopped buying Art. I made the "cause" to borrow money from one of my wealthy patrons to alleviate this stress.

I had also stress from emotional problems when a man I believed I was in love with ran off to marry one of his old girlfriends. I made the "cause" to get into therapy to help me get through the subsequent depression I fell into.

I had been overeating, especially meat. This was a desperate attempt to fill the lonely vacuum in my life as a result of losing my boyfriend. I made the "cause" to go off meat and dairy products, underrating for a month to clean out my colon. Instead of these high-fat, fibreless foods, I substituted carrot juice, orange juice, lots of raw and lightly cooked vegetables and fruits, whole grains, fish, nuts, and herbs to clean out and detoxify my body paving the way back to health.

Because of my depression, I had let my exercise routine deteriorate into sitting in the hot tub at the gym, feeling sorry for myself. I made the "cause" to swim one mile, five days a week at the YMCA.

USE SPIRITUALITY IN YOUR EVERYDAY LIFE

You can transform any illness with spirituality. Using prayer and reviewing "causes" can get you in touch with the reality of your situation and show a path for transformation. Chanting and praying creates healing energy. Combined with visualization, seeing yourself transformed into health as you pray, for instance, you have a most powerful healing tool.

Interest in spirituality and healing has moved to the forefront. Harvard Medical School hosted a conference on spirituality and health, focusing on the healing effects of forgiveness. A tremendous shift in the medical profession's openness to the subject is taking place.

Be determined to regain your health if you have lost it! Prayer can help you. Visualize yourself happy and doing what makes you happiest as you pray or chant. Helping others will also manifest healing energy, so include a plan in your visualization. Cancer cells are very self-centered. When you help others, you begin to change the nature of those cells.

The amazing transformation of my Cancer from a weak, anemic pitiful state to one of glowing health and no tumors amazed my Doctor. He was so impressed he joined the YMCA himself! We exercised together. I would catch him looking at me in such a strange way, as if I were a reincarnated ghost or Dead Woman Exercising! He had predicted he would soon be attending my funeral, but only two months later, I was standing at the gym in tights and a leotard pumping iron!

Although it did take me seven more months of staying religiously on the MOTEP program to regain the healthy state I enjoy today.

CANCER IS A SPIRITUAL DISEASE

Cancer is first and foremost a spiritual disease. It is always a *systemic* disease, involving the spirit, the mind, and the body. While a toxic body condition has to be cleaned out, the transformation into health requires spiritual strength. Hope, expectation, and determination will reactivate a sluggish immune system. Trust in the body's wisdom will activate the healing systems. Forgiveness will release stress and blocks that cause tumors to grow.

Prayer, chanting and visualization create the true healing energy that high-tech equipment and cutting-edge treatments can never match. Use your heartfelt, deep spiritual strength to reclaim your highest level of health. Use your spiritual practice daily and combine it with imaginative, powerful visualizations, and health will follow slowly but surely. You can pray to reverse a "terminal" diagnosis and win. Amaze your doctors whose look of incredulity, disbelief and shock will be worth the whole effort.

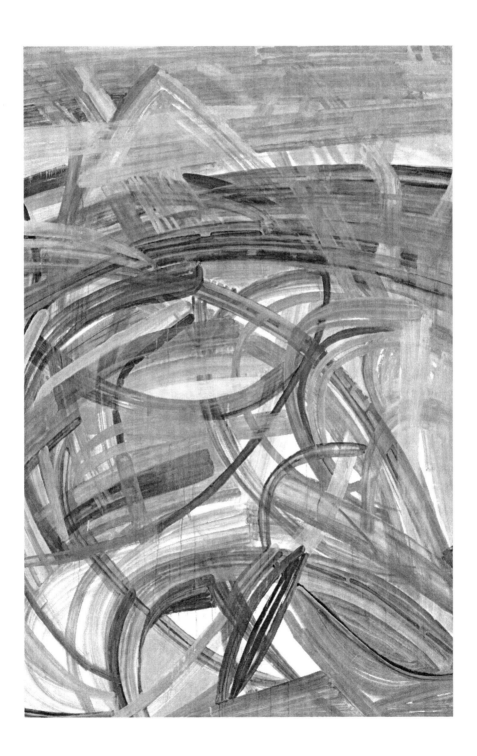

CHAPTER 17

The Healing Power of Group Therapy

AS AN ART and Psychology major at the University of Nevada, I have gained insight into how important psychosocial support can be in healing trauma and disease. My Master's Degree work in the area of suicide also gave me many clues. In 1967, Dr. James B. Nichols was my instructor and partner when I obtained a grant in psychology. He asked me what area I would like to explore. As he had just taught a class I took on the subject of suicide, I suggested we do research in the local area we lived in—Reno, Nevada.

To our astonishment, Nevada turned out to have the highest suicide rate in the nation! This was a significant finding and surprised us. We decided there and then to start a Suicide Prevention Center. We enlisted the help of Norman Farbarow and Edward Schneidman who had begun a call-in Suicide Prevention Center in Los Angeles. We invited them to Reno to give a lecture, then picked their brains. We used the pattern they had established to start our own center. I am happy to report that this Suicide Prevention Center in Reno is still in operation today, forty-one years later!

We decided to do research, visiting the homes of a long list of people who had made a suicide attempt that had been documented. This was instructive. Certain characteristics began to emerge, so visiting these homes began to have a familiar ring. It was almost as if we visited one home, with subtle differences, in various locations!

The characteristic that stood out above all others was the totally reclusive nature of these environments. There was something "shut in" and off-putting about these homes that often displayed warnings against visitors, such as "BEWARE OF THE DOG," "NO SOLICITORS," "DO NOT DISTURB," or other paranoid tinged warnings. There was something closed-off and secretive about these people. The few times that we would get them to open the door, they appeared angrily hesitant, and almost grudgingly would utter a word. We saw only a part of their face peering warily out as if we were the Sheriff coming to arrest them! "What do you want?" they would often curtly demand.

We had prepared a survey, but few of these people would take the time to answer questions. They appeared very disturbed by having visitors and felt threatened. They made it perfectly clear that we were totally unwelcome and often shut the door in our face!

HOSTILITY IN SUICIDAL PERSONS

The hostility we faced was unexpected. Reno is a neighborly town. As a young Girl Scout, I had sold, one cold winter, miniature clear plastic Christmas trees, decorated with tiny colored glass spheres in brilliant gem-like colors that I wired onto the trees myself. I made a bundle, talking to neighbors, many of whom I didn't even know. Some had even invited me inside to warm up and to display my wares, or shared their Christmas cookie baking with me. I related to my Mother the kindness and friendliness I had encountered on my sales route, making the job easy and enjoyable.

But these people were far different!

I began to see that the striking characteristic of many people who had been suicidal was a distinct hostility and loneliness that they seemed to foster. In times of extreme depression, when life seemed unbearable, they, in all probability, had no one to turn to or talk to about their problems. Perhaps that is why the Suicide Prevention Center became such a brilliant success in Reno. Now there was a telephone number that these closed and shut-in people could anonymously call to do the important work of getting their feelings out!

Years later, I came to the realization that Cancer might be a form of passive suicide, however subconscious.

NIGELLA'S MOTHER AND HUSBAND GET Cancer

Nigella Lawson, the cookbook goddess from England, is a stunningly beautiful, but modest woman whom I met at her book signing recently. When Nigella was twenty-five, a doctor found that her mother, Vanessa, had Liver Cancer. He gave her the prognosis of only a few months more to live. He suggested that Nigella break the news.

"It was very hard," Nigella says. "I think she wasn't a particularly happy woman, so there was a part of her that didn't want to live." Together, they wrote the death announcement.

"You better put down it was Cancer, because people will think it was suicide," Vanessa instructed her. "And, of course, you and I know that it is."

Vanessa called the undertaker herself to order the type of coffin she wanted.

"And what is the name of the deceased?" the undertaker inquired.

"It's me," Vanessa replied merrily.

"She was nearing the end of her forty-eighth year and very, very grateful she hadn't gone into her forty-ninth when she died," her daughter sighed.

Nigella's personal interest in Cancer escalated when her husband, John Diamond, a columnist, became ill with Throat Cancer. "As he became sicker, he turned into someone other than himself," Nigella relates. "A complete living nightmare. Because he was unhappy and angry, quite, rightly furious, he blamed me. Yes, he was angry at me. Well, not at me, you know, but I was the one to do it to." She hardly knew him anymore. "He really hated to be this person so full of anger and bitterness. He was having his life taken away. It was torturing him."

Nigella was very interested in learning more about Cancer. In both these cases, I believe a regular group therapy session would have helped both her mother and her husband. Perhaps a group of women could have helped Vanessa find reasons to live. Maybe John Diamond could have found a way to vent some of the anger that was building up inside of him exacerbating his Cancer. It definitely would have helped his relationship with Nigella, had he been able to release some of his anger in a group therapy session, instead of taking out all his hostility and frustration on her!

CLINICAL STUDIES SHOW GROUP THERAPY HELPS HEAL

Dr. David Spiegel at Stanford University paved the way, showing the dramatic results of group therapy in Breast Cancer patients. He did not set out to show longer survival, but set up a group therapy weekly session for terminally ill Breast Cancer patients to reduce anxiety and depression and improve coping skills. Dr. Spiegel was stunned by his 1977 study, when he reviewed it years later. Two women survived and one lived until 1990! Compared to those who did not participate, the women in the group sessions lived twice as long.

"Social support seems to be one factor that shows up again and again that seems to influence many different illnesses," writes Steven Locke, author of the book, *The Healer Within.*

Dr. Spiegel goes even further to say that, "Frankly, group support may have a more powerful effect than many of the other physical interventions we do. I believe group therapy should be a part of the recovery plan for any major illness. Having a support group to share pain, laughter and tears is a very powerful thing."

In further observations, Dr. Spiegel noted that male Cancer patients did better if they were married, while women survived longer if they retained strong ties to *women* friends.

GROUP THERAPY HELPED ME TO CONQUER MY CANCER

It is not necessary to join a group specific for Cancer. The group I joined was simply a get-together of women, a pot-luck where we brought a homemade dish and sat in a circle talking about our lives. In fact no one in the group, at first, knew I was fighting Breast and Uterine Cancer. I would put on make-up, dress nicely, and bring my dish. I presented a façade of normalcy.

However, the secret came out one night when we did highly prophetic Rune Cards. Supposedly, they were done just for fun, entertainment, and a change of pace. I did not know the wisdom of the Runes or their uncanny ability to predict the future! These fortune –teller cards are ancient, going all the way back to the Vikings. I approached this pastime with extreme trepidation! I had enjoyed the company and the dinner. I was reluctant, however, to talk about my extreme health crisis.

But the Rune cards can't be fooled. We were to draw two giant cards apiece. The first card I chose was a beautiful illustration of two swans, their long necks lovingly entwined. The explanation was that I would soon have a partner. The single women in the group sighed wistfully and nodded approval.

The next card, however, was a shock! It depicted a glaringly lit hospital operating room with a long, empty white operating platform over which a surgeon in a white mask, head-covering and latex gloves loomed menacingly. The caption was "The patient on the operating table is you!" The women later related that I had turned white and mute! On the back the explanation was that I had something in my life that needed excising. The advice was "Operate on yourself!"

I was so very glad to have the support of a friendly, warm group of women. The cards offered a confession I did not have to verbalize. I could only sit there, stunned. The group, somehow recognizing I was in shock at this uncanny experience, tactfully moved on to the next subject.

On the long drive home over the freeways, I chanted "Operate on Yourself" over and over.

A MEDICALLY ORIENTED GROUP THAT
REPULSED CHERYL CANFIELD

Cheryl Canfield disliked the medically oriented group she attended. She writes:

"I entered a large room where tables had been pushed together end-to-end to form a rectangle. As I slid into the cold metal chair, quizzical faces nodded and smiled in my direction. Swollen, pale, the faces were captivating. One was especially thin under the dome of a baldhead. My eyes glanced at the hands that were wrapped around cans of Coke and Pepsi. In the middle of the table was a large square cake, the white frosting thick and dotted with sugary flowers of pink, yellow, and green. Plates of cookies lined both sides.

"I was tremendously moved by the struggles of the individuals sitting around the table, but I couldn't relate to the unquestioning acceptance that the attending physician's opinion was the only one that mattered. No one seemed to question the treatments that were recommended or consider diet or lifestyle changes or to factor in the effect of emotions on their disease. There was no mention of how Cancer feeds on the kind of sugary treats that decorated the table.

"I was especially bothered by what seemed to be the view that Cancer is a random event that attacks certain victims for no particular reason and that there is nothing we can personally do about it."

Cheryl becomes even more committed to meeting Cancer her own way. "I was determined not to be a victim," she writes. She decided to heal herself completely and naturally "one step at a time."

Meeting Cheryl at a book signing some years after her self-healing, I was struck by her glowing health, her shiny hair, and her quiet but determined demeanor. She impressed me as someone who had a very strong inner fortitude.

SOCIAL SUPPORT CRUCIAL IN CANCER HEALING

The most important factor in group therapy seems to be social support. The group you gather around you, or the group you attend need not be Cancer-specific for you to obtain benefit and healing energy. Support groups should bolster one's desire to get well.

There are two well-established psychosocial Cancer support groups you can check out. The **Wellness Community** in California and **Gilda's Club** in New York both offer Cancer patients group therapy sessions. Both these organizations are expanding into other states, so consult your phone book to see if there is one near you. They offer a variety of group support and programs that will help you to regain your sense of control and well-being.

Harold Benjamin and Norman Cousins started the Wellness Community. Gilda Radner was one of their first clients!

I attended an Orientation Meeting for the Wellness Community that was led by Jan, a twelve-year survivor of a difficult Cancer that had begun in her brain. She now had a tumor wrapped around her right retina that left her with one working eye. Her right eye was swollen closed. Yet she astounded me with her enthusiasm and zest for life. She was joking about her new glasses that were so obnoxious that they dumbfounded the clerk at the license bureau into renewing her driver's license! Apparently he didn't see her right eye that clearly through her dark glasses. She can still drive, only having problems parking because of loss of stereovision. She has submitted to numerous surgeries and multiple radiation treatments to her face that have eliminated her salivary glands. She must constantly drink water.

Though no Medical treatment has worked to stop her Cancer, nothing has stopped her courageous spirit from taking joy in every day life. She does Tai Chi, swims, walks and leads groups at the Wellness Community in Pasadena. "This community helped save my life!" she enthuses. She is a world traveler having gone to her son's wedding in India and taking exotic vacations. She is adamant that the disease should not stop your parties and celebrations. "Don't put your life on hold," she admonished. "Trees bend in strong winds, but they do not fall down."

The first time that I had called the Wellness Community, (years ago when writing my first book), they told me they required participants to go through the Medical treatment before attending their events and classes. Times have changed! They now let people participate who are doing only Alternative treatments.

"It's your body," Jan pointed out. *"You make the decisions."*

Jan made me feel very welcome. I later attended a lecture on Chinese Medicine there that I will describe in a later chapter.

If you seek out a group you feel comfortable with, it will help you on your road back to health. The life you save could be your own!

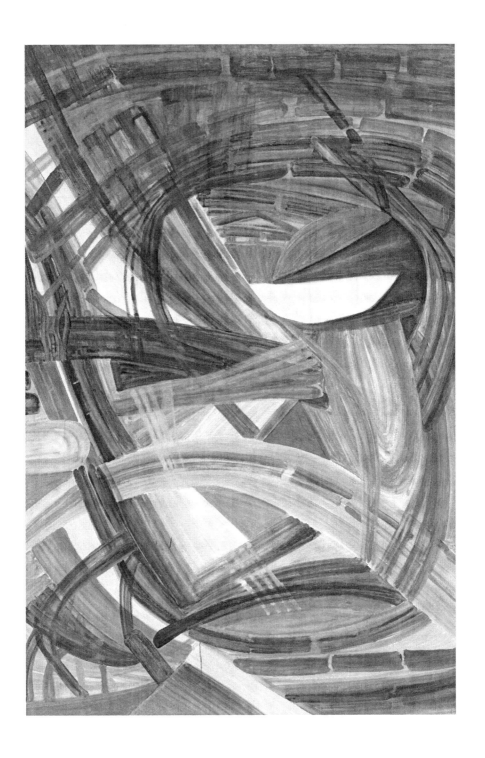

CHAPTER 18

Making The Decisions

WHEN FACED WITH a diagnosis of any form of Cancer, it is easy to become terrified. The doctor is telling you point blank that the monstrous disease you have could be terminal. You probably have had friends or relatives who died of Cancer. After the initial shock, you might still feel a tremendous amount of overwhelming fear and anxiety.

But this is not the time to panic. Rather it is a time when you will be questioning, trying to decide on options about how to proceed. Also you must face the pivotal, central question, "Do you want to live?"

If the answer is "no," please do my "lucky exercise." List the ten things you feel lucky to have. Do this every day until you see how fortunate you are to be among the living. Life is the greatest gift, and that gift has been bestowed upon you to use it anyway you see fit. It's up to you to create a happy life. If you are unhappy, what steps can you take to make your life more serene? Find a way to validate your existence!

YES, I WANT TO LIVE

If the answer is "yes," you are in much better shape, especially if it is a resounding affirmation of your life. However, you still must make important decisions; now you must plan your route back to health.

The doctor may pressure you to begin surgery, chemotherapy, radiation, and/or hormone treatments. These will be described as "traditional," "standard," "conventional," or "routine." These words are reassuring sales terms! He has no cure to offer you. Even a new gene treatment or clinical trial can offer no guarantees that it will help you to get well.

"Let the buyer beware," has never been so apropos!

As Dr. Susan Love, a breast surgeon and health researcher emphasizes, do not be in a big hurry to yield to pressure! Generally, this is not a huge emergency that must be radically and aggressively treated immediately! In all probability, it took years to acquire your disease. You still have time to make your decision based on second opinions, research on the Internet, books, and talking to others who have been through Cancer or are knowledgeable. You may want to go on the MOTEP program for two- to- four months, as quite a lot of progress can be made in that short period of time. You will start on the road to reversing your condition. After four months, if you do the program with all your sincerity, energy, and heartfelt focus, you will see tremendous progress. You can go back to your doctor for more tests. You are then in the driver's seat to make decisions whether you want to continue rebuilding your health or submit to some or all of the Medical Treatment.

The doctors may try to intimidate you with their statistics and threats that the "the Cancer may spread." However, the very instant you put faith in your own body's plentiful resources, is the minute you will initiate the healing processes. In my experience and that of many others, most of the problems and symptoms can be cleared up within the four months on the MOTEP program. You will at least see much improvement.

Although I don't recommend an instant "cure," Belinda cleared her problem mammogram in only ten days on the program! Take four months to detoxify and de-stress your mind and your body. This will often be enough time to reverse your symptoms. However, if you are like me, it will then take the rest of the year to thoroughly rebuild your health so that you feel normal.

Instead of the attitude implied by the book on Breast Cancer, *Just Get Me Through It,* take some time out to really reflect on your life and options.

REVIEW YOUR LIFE

Review your life to see what effects exposure to carcinogens, caffeine, over-eating, overweight, lack of an exercise program, conflicted relationships, depression from overwhelming stresses such as deaths of loved ones, divorce, or separation have had on you.

Try to find new ways of dealing with financial stress, relationships, and hardships in your life. See if you are "on your path," doing what you always wanted to do, at least part time. Remember when one door closes, another opens. Use **defeat as a springboard** to your next major success! This is the secret of life.

DISEASE CANNOT BE POISONED OUT OF THE BODY

The Medical System cannot cut, poison, or burn Cancer out of your body! This paradigm is a fantasy and eventually must give way to a whole body-mind-spirit healing.

The idea of poisoning disease out of the body is not new. In fact it is antiquated. In the book *Nature Cures—The History of Alternative Medicine,* James C. Whorton writes about this absurd idea.

In the 1800s', the standard therapy for most any disease was a medicine called Calomel. It was the most frequently prescribed drug of the time, given to most patients just as antibiotics are so commonly prescribed today.

"This was a powerful cathartic that physicians believed would flush morbid material from the body while also stimulating the liver to greater action. But as a mercury compound (mercurous chloride), calomel was toxic, and when given in repeated doses over a period of days or weeks, it made the patient's mouth painfully swollen, causing cheeks and gums to bleed and ulcerate and teeth to become loose and fall out. In severe cases, the sufferer's jawbone could be destroyed. All too often, critics charged, the mercurial treatment left the sick maimed and disfigured, subjects of pity and horror." Such injuries were compounded by ptyalism, a profuse flow of viscous, foul-smelling saliva streaming out at the rate from a pint to a quart in twenty-four hours.

"This was considered proof that an adequate dose was given. Doctors then rationalized the side effects as necessary evils, much as oncologists today justify the damages done by Cancer chemotherapy. Thus the doctors saw the risks being outweighed by the "benefits," from such ghastly and toxic treatment.

"Patients, understandably, dreaded a course of calomel treatment and submitted to it as an evil almost as formidable as the disease for which it was administered. Yet the great majority did submit!"

Other standard and conventional treatments of the time included bloodletting, the infamous treatment that killed George Washington, often with leaches to remove the patient's "bad blood." These treatments were referred to as "heroic" therapy!

REGULAR VS. IRREGULAR DOCTORS

While calomel treatments were prescribed by the regular doctors, there were irregular doctors who enlisted the mind to heal the body. In the late 1700s, Franz Anton Mesmer experimented with "mind cures," using magnets at first, then gradually utilizing the power of hypnosis (the term "to mesmerize" originated with him). He had dramatic results with many patients, even with tumors. He believed that a patient must go through a crisis, sometimes violent, in order to heal. "A disease cannot be healed without a crisis," he stated. Mesmer helped the patient create the healing crisis using the imagination of the patient along with the power of his own suggestion.

His work influenced other "irregular" healers such as Charles Poyen, who introduced magnetic healing to America in 1835. He attempted to convince George Washington to try the new method of healing, but was, unfortunately for George, unsuccessful. The whole history of our country might have been rewritten had he been able to convince President Washington that conventional bloodletting was not the best method of healing disease!

In the early 1800s, Phineas Quimby offered a "Mind Cure." He was noted to cure a man who couldn't walk or speak and another who was unable to lift his arm for two years. He employed an assistant who, when hypnotized, could diagnose and prescribe herbs for almost any patient he turned his subconscious attention to! After many years of success, Quimby decided that "Cure therefore should be simply a matter of *identifying and correcting a patient's negative beliefs,* replacing them with a positive state of mind, the body would be freed to function properly and overcome its pathology." He instilled faith into his clients, convinced them they were healthy, by talking them through their negative thoughts one-by-one.

A man who had been confined to bed for four years summoned Quimby. "Mr. Quimby commenced taking up his feelings, one by one, like a lawyer examining witnesses, analyzing them and showing him he had put false constructions on all his feelings." The patient, Robinson, thought his logic "so plain that it was impossible not to understand." He subsequently woke the next day, got out of bed, and felt well, leading a normal life from that day forward.

One patient who came to see Quimby was an extremely ill woman named Mary Baker Patterson. Her second husband had sent her to see him. In her subsequent healing, she became a prophet. Over the next seven years, she taught healing according to his principles and wrote "Key to the Scriptures." Upon marrying her third husband, Gilbert Eddy, Mary Baker Eddy built her foundation in Christian Science, using the mind and spirit to heal disease instead of the drugs and surgery that the "regular" doctors used. She had astounding success creating her new healing religion, donating two million dollars to her church upon her death. Today her multitude of followers practice self-healing using prayer.

MAKE DECISIONS CAREFULLY

Conventional methods of treating Cancer have only been "standard" for about one hundred years in over four thousand years that medicine has been practiced. These methods have never been "proven to be effective." According to the survey in the book, *Our Bodies, Ourselves*, when you look at the lifetime of the individual with Cancer as opposed to the short five-year period considered by the Medical Establishment as the "cure rate," eighty percent will die with or from their disease.

Your doctor might tell you that because they caught your particular Cancer early, there is a "ninety-five percent cure rate." But this percentage is misleading because it only represents the people with the type of Cancer you have who have not recurred for five years after diagnosis and does not include recurrences or other types of Cancer or health problems they may have encountered from their treatments. The fact is, as everyone knows, there is no "cure" for Cancer. So how can there be a "cure rate?"

"There are lies, damn lies, and statistics in that order," Mark Twain wryly observed. When considering only a short period of time after treatment, statistics can be shuffled and shifted to make treatments look effective, when in fact they are often only temporary, leading to the terms "remission" and "recurrence." Also Medical Treatments are carcinogenic leading to further Cancers down the road. Surgery creates scar tissue upping the chance of Cancer in that area. Chemotherapy suppresses the immune system opening up the body to further disease and even more Cancer. Often the patient dies of "complications" from Cancer treatment rather than from the disease itself!

Radiation has been proven to be extremely carcinogenic from Hiroshima to Love Canal. Radiation, as reported by John Robbins in his book, *Reclaiming Your Health*, became part of Cancer treatment at the turn of the Century. A man named William Douglas who owned Uranium mines offered to donate a large amount of money to Memorial Sloan Kettering Cancer Hospital in New York providing they would use his Uranium in their Cancer treatment! In accepting the grant, they somehow overlooked the obvious fact that radiation *causes* Cancer.

Radiation is high-speed atomic particles that destroy any part of the body at which they are aimed. Genetic mutations and cell aberration can result from exposure. Cumulative damage can occur throughout the body. One of the "side effects" of Cancer treatment with radiation is further Cancer years later, a case of today's treatment becoming tomorrow's disease. In Breast Cancer, seriously burned lungs can result leading to death because the patient is unable to breathe. Heart damage from the radiation has also been showing up twelve to twenty years after this treatment.

But why submit to mutilation, poisoning and dangerous

radiation when a detoxification program with high-energy exercise and spiritual support over the following four months might work just as well or better to start you back on the road to health?

RISKS OF SURGERY

In his book, *Complications—A Surgeon's Notes on an Imperfect Science*, Atul Gawande admits, "Even with the simplest operation, it cannot be taken for granted that a patient will come through better off—or even alive."

Medical error in surgery can begin in the first stage while putting a patient asleep. An eighteen-year old perfectly healthy young woman went to the hospital to have her wisdom teeth pulled under general anesthesia. The anesthesiologist inserted the breathing tube into her esophagus instead of her trachea which is a relatively common mishap as they are very close together. Failing to spot the error, the patient, deprived of oxygen, died. Mistakes, Gawande recounts, are an inevitable part of medicine.

Olivia Goldsmith, author of the book, *First Wives Club* that was made into a movie, was a character. I met her at the Governor's Conference where she was to speak when Sharon Stone cancelled out. We both had a laugh about this. Olivia was talented and a persuasive speaker, a strong woman, but hardly beautiful. She didn't seem self-conscious about her looks. I would never have guessed that a couple of years later she would die of the anesthesia given for her cosmetic plastic surgery operation!

The *Journal of the American Medical Association* recorded

that iatrogenic disease (caused by doctors) is the third leading cause of disease after Heart Disease and Cancer! Drugs
account for the biggest segment of Medical Malpractice suits,
not only for the wrong dose or the wrong prescription, but
also for the *correct* dosage of the prescribed medication!

Disease cannot be cut out of the body. Surgery for Cancer
is not always the magic cure we have hoped for.

CANCER IS NEVER A LOCAL DISEASE

When my friend Kimberly, age thirty-four, found a lump
in her breast, she submitted to a mastectomy. The mammogram had been negative, but they did a biopsy that showed
Cancer. So three days later her beautiful breast was ampu-
tated. However, the Cancer recurred.

Where it returned woke me from my "Santa Claus" notion
that disease can be cut out of the body.

Kimberly's Breast Cancer recurred in the very same spot,
the chest wall where her breast used to be!

Later I found out that this "loco-regional recurrence"
happens regularly, in as many as one-third of Breast Cancer
operations. *The Cancer returns in same area.*

I learned then and there that *Cancer is always a systemic disease*. It cannot be surgically removed from one
area of the body.

Kimberly submitted to so much Chemotherapy and Radiation she no longer had an immune system. She caught every
cold and flu going around. Two broken rib bones resulted
from all the radiation they subjected her to. The Autologous
Bone-Marrow Transplant she submitted to almost killed
her. Although a strong fighter who believed in the Medical

and followed all their rules and prescriptions, she died at age thirty-eight, a week after her birthday, an emaciated, ill, and broken young woman.

I believe the Medical Treatments, not the Cancer, killed her. The anger I felt at the barbaric, destructive and toxic treatments she received fueled the drive I had to write my first book on Breast Cancer.

MAKING THE RIGHT DECISIONS

When making decisions about Cancer, please be very careful. I believe the present standard treatment is archaic and will be evolving into Alternative Medicine soon. Eighty-five percent of Cancer patients already use some form of Alternative Medicine. We are in a new age of enlightened mind-body healing. The Medical Establishment is even interested, coining a long, difficult name for it—Psychoneuroimmunology—or PNI.

Old ways die hard. Surgeons were initially reluctant to give up mastectomies even when they found lumpectomies achieved the exact same results. Full breast radiation was used, but recent studies show that doing only local radiation produced the exact same results.

The economic incentive to do "standard treatment" is very strong. Insurance companies pay more for mastectomies than lumpectomies.

For all the sacrifice of amputation, poisoning with chemotherapy, and burning with radiation, the Medical Establishment cannot offer you a "cure." They cannot even guarantee any benefits from these brutal treatments.

G.K. Roumani, M.D. suggests that the patient and his

family should question their doctors when any proposed treatment is offered for Prostate Cancer: Are there other options for me? What if I do not treat this Cancer? What is the expected quality of life after treatment? What are the side effects of the treatment? And always get a second opinion. (*Los Angeles Times* Aug 9, 2008).

YOU CAN HEAL FROM CANCER NATURALLY

You can heal from Cancer step-by-step, day-by-day by building your body up instead of destroying it with Medical Treatment. Make a commitment to get well. When you plan your route back to health, consider everything. Make your decisions carefully. The life you save may be your own!

CHAPTER 19

Energy Healing

WHAT'S A NICE Jewish girl like you doing in Chinatown? I wondered to myself. I had gone to a Chinese doctor and was eating Chinese food at my favorite restaurant for Oriental food when this thought popped into my head.

I had never been to an Acupuncturist. The idea of sticking needles into my skin had, frankly, never been all that appealing. Acupuncture is now an accepted alternative in Cancer treatment. How could I write about something I have never tried?

But then the accident happened. Overtired one day, I pulled down the heavy wooden garage door of my studio on my foot. I doubled over in intense pain!

The next week I went nowhere. I couldn't even walk! Because of the immense swelling, no shoe fit on my left foot that was a hot red balloon before it turned black, deep purple, dark green and other macabre colors. Putting a pillow under my lower leg so the foot didn't touch the sheets or have the pressure of my body upon it was the only way to sleep. I experienced unrelenting, searing pain!

After a week of being an invalid, I could finally go to the YMCA, but only for my fifty-minute swim, hot tub and sauna. Mary, a Korean, immediately noticed my foot in the locker room and exclaimed, "You should do acupuncture! It will heal so much faster—four or five days! You should go at the first sign of pain. Go today!"

I figured it was worth a try. In the phone book I found Dr. Jane Chan in Chinatown. She was able to make an appointment for me later that afternoon.

I could drive using mostly my right foot. I entered limping. She gave me some forms to fill out as I noticed her office could use a coat of white paint and some cleaning up. I decided to ignore the mess. Pain offers a lot of motivation.

She asked me questions about my injury and put me on her table. Deciding my foot needed at least six needles, I almost panicked. My foot was too tender to even touch. She was going to stick six needles into it?!

ACUPUNCTURE WORKS

Dr.Chan pulled out what looked like a matchbook that opened revealing very fine needles. With some antiseptic, she swabbed my foot at various points and then stuck in the needles. It wasn't too bad. However, when she thought she needed a seventh needle, I objected vociferously.

She settled for six and put clamps on the needles as if she were jump-starting a car battery. She turned on a machine generating electricity. At the same time she turned on a heat lamp aiming it at my sore foot. A timer was set for twenty minutes. I began to feel a mild vibration inside my foot. Grin and bear it is my motto. Twenty minutes seemed like a long time. But the butterfly fluttering of the electricity began to feel good. When the timer rang, I actually was enjoying the warm fluttering. She then removed the needles, which wasn't as painful as I thought it would be. She rubbed some herb oil that smelled a bit like Eucalyptus on my foot.

"No one could touch your foot when you came in," she reminded me. Now she was able to massage it with the oil. I felt no pain! She then put patches of herbs on my foot, giving me some extra for the next day.

I realized I had had a form of energy healing.

I asked her about treatment for Cancer. She said Cancer patients came in, mainly for alleviation of pain. She described the gastrointestinal damage she saw from Chemotherapy. She had never heard of Self-Lumpectomy or self-healing Cancer, but she was very interested.

Feeling ravenous, I hobbled to my favorite Chinese restaurant. My foot burned and was as hot as a stove. Finally, it turned cool, like an ice cube.

Sleeping that night, my foot was again hot. In the morning I awoke and stepped on my foot. Miraculously, there was no pain. I wasn't limping either. At the gym I noticed that the black color had turned to mostly pink again. I was now a convert to acupuncture

ANOUSH HEALS WITH HIS ENERGY

In my book on Breast Cancer, I described Anoush who lashed out his arm as if recharging it, then circled a baby with a kidney tumor who was sleeping face down on her Mother's lap. Circling his arm over the baby without actually touching her, the baby jerked up. This seemed like something out of a new-wave science-fiction movie. I could actually feel the energy as if the whole room was plugged into the wall-socket. This was my introduction to energy healing.

When it was my turn, I explained to Anoush that I had just done Self-Lumpectomy on two tumors. I was there only to interview him. He began to interview me, as he had never heard of Self-Lumpectomy!

He asked where my breast tumor had been located. I challenged him to find it.

Using his arm as his diagnostic tool, he began circling my chest area. First one breast and then the other. He did not ask me to remove my heavy cotton tunic outfit with a long sweater. He went around and around. Finally he came to one spot. "It was there," he stated.

"How did you know?" I asked amazed. He had found the *exact* spot!

"The spot was "heavy," he told me. He then looked frightened for me and asked if he might do a complete exam.

I stood in shock as he went over my body, top to bottom, using only his arm, not touching me, circling in wide arcs. I felt his magnetic energy as he made his rounds. He then told me that my thyroid was "heavy" as was my right ovary and left kidney. He then looked terrified. "You're lucky!" he exclaimed.

Luck, I told him, was definitely with me. But also I had put myself on a crash health program covering every aspect of my life.

I asked him what he meant by the term "heavy."

"The acupuncture meridians are blocked. The flow of energy, or Chi, as the life force is called in Chinese medicine was blocked and had gotten stuck at certain points resulting in tumors," he explained.

This made sense. Crossing my arms across my breasts and crossing my legs at the same time I tensed my body with financial and emotional turmoil and stress. This had, I suddenly realized, contributed to the formation of the two tumors.

When he finished the exam, I felt refreshed, as if I had just emerged from a spring-water pool. The dose of energy had transformed me. That night I slept like a rock!

Anoush explained that after a long fall when climbing mountains, he had discovered he had healing energy while in the hospital. He sought to develop his newfound ability further by studying with a healer. He claimed he could heal others using only his energy field. He had vanquished a tumor in his own wife's breast, for instance, and he had many other examples.

USING YOUR OWN HANDS TO HEAL

But there are still more surprises to come! **You can use your own hands to help your body to heal!** In the book, *Your Hands Can Heal You*, Master Stephen Co and Eric B. Robins, M.D. with John Merryman describe how you can utilize the healing electric energy your own body generates to heal yourself and others. The method is termed "Pranic Healing." I utilized these exercises on my foot to increase healing and alleviate pain. Prana is another word for "life force." To do this kind of healing, an open mind and a positive attitude must be maintained.

YOUR ENERGETIC ANATOMY

Both Acupuncture and Pranic healing are based on the theory that you have an energetic anatomy, just as you have a physical anatomy. Illnesses and injuries appear in the energetic anatomy before they appear in the physical one. **Your body has an innate ability to repair itself.** Just as forming a scab, while the white blood cells underneath the scab build new tissue will repair a skinned knee, your body can rebuild and repair most any injury or disease it is threatened by. Doctors know that this happens, but they don't know how the body does this, or what force powers the efforts. Though traditional medical thinking assumes this healing is beyond our willful control, Prana healing teaches that we can harness healing energy and direct it to help an injury or illness return to normal.

Through life force generating exercises, Qi or chi can be built up. Reiki is a Japanese energy-channeling system of massage. There is also Therapeutic Touch. In India the art is call Ayurveda, a form of natural energy healing. Yoga practices also incorporate spiritual energy to heal.

In Pranic healing you use white and colored energy with your hands to "sweep" the body, clearing the blockages. Both Chakras, various parts of your body, and auras—the energy pattern surrounding you—are involved. Meridians are the body's energy channels, used to put the needles in when practicing acupuncture.

The three main sources of prana energy are the air, the earth, and the sun. We get this energy from respiration, through our feet touching the earth as we walk, and the sun that also feeds us indirectly from the food we eat. Your prana can be diminished or weakened by many factors: your beliefs, emotions, attitudes, inhibitions, traumatic memories, food you eat, people you associate with, where you live and work, how you work and live, what you say, what you think, and how you react to the stress level you encounter in your daily life. When your prana is low or dirty, you typically experience some type of health problem.

Pranic healing starts with deep breathing exercises. You then build up energy with your hands. You announce your intention to heal certain parts of your body by looking at them and holding your hand slightly above that part. You then sweep and move above the part, visualizing a white or blue-green light, for instance, emanating from your hands. Different colors help different problems. Electric violet is good for almost any pain, injury or disease.

Thus others' energy or your own energy can be utilized to help make you well and free of pain.

CHINESE MEDICINE AND ENERGY HEALING

At the Wellness Community, Lucy Postolov, L.Ac., a Russian doctor who spent several years studying Chinese Medicine, gave a workshop. She pointed out that there is not "one tool" to "kill Cancer." "The Chinese have a different view of tumors and Cancer," she explained.

In Chinese Medicine, Cancer is always tied to the emotions. Every organ connects up to certain emotions. Lung Cancer is usually tied to grief. Breast Cancer is believed to be manifested from problems with a husband, a sister-in-law, or mother-in-law! A hardened area in the breast would turn to stone. The source of this information dates back five thousand years to the time of the Yellow Emperor. The goal in treatment was to detoxify the body and then build up immunity. Emotions are always worked on. They are considered the trigger points for all Cancers.

Forgiveness and letting go of resentments and emotional pain are essential psychological steps in healing.

Moving energy into blocked Meridian channels is accomplished with intention and movement: acupuncture, acupressure, exercises like Tai Chi and Chi Gong, and meditation. There are Meridian channels throughout the body, one-hundred-fifty points in the ear alone! You can affect every organ through the ear. There are fifteen hundred acupuncture points. Every one of these points, interestingly enough, has a connection to the brain.

Acupuncture stimulates endorphin response. Endorphins are chemicals released from the brain when we feel joy.

Chinese Medicine emphasizes the power of stomach breathing (the stomach goes out with each inhale of oxygen and back in upon exhale), and meditation. The issue of what organ is out of balance is addressed. Tai Chi teaches the movement of energy through simple, beautiful movements to achieve harmony and balance.

Here I remembered watching Tai Chi being performed at sunset around a beautiful mineral-water swimming pool surrounded by deep-purple mountains in the warm, dry air of Desert Hot Springs. A rhythmic dance in slow motion, coordinating two participants in graceful harmony, this exercise was a beautiful slow dance, a ritual to the Gods of Healing.

There is also a balance between giving and receiving. This issue needs to be addressed. In order to keep energy open and free flowing, the balance needs to be equalized. Everything in the Universe is connected.

A Chinese Proverb is that "a worm won't enter a growing tree." This applies to Cancer in many ways. When we "get stuck" in our lives, our energy gets blocked and we feel stagnated, our cells also get stuck. The immune system stops working at full force and we might be diagnosed with Candida or other parasites. Cancer, to the Chinese way of thinking, means you must **"change everything you did before."**

Cancer has a low vibration. To increase your vibration you do exercise. Yoga or Tai Chi is included in Chinese Cancer treatment. In my case I did fifty minutes of swimming five days a week.

Find out why you are in a low vibrational mode and change that state with high-intensity workouts. You can also change that vibration with high-energy action and finding a new direction for your life. **Enthusiasm for getting up in the morning is essential to health.**

The Chinese view of Cancer, in my view, comes closer to the truth than our Western way of looking only at tumors or blood-cell counts. Chinese look at the emotions, energy and diet of the patient. They heal with herbs, nutrition, exercise, and by removing psychological and emotional blocks to getting well. They have the patient look hard at their lifestyle and remove self-destructive practices.

The patient then, is not a robot with a tumor, but a person with emotional conflicts and blocked energy who must make the effort and take the time to change his or her life. They must do healing exercises, take herbs, go on a special diet, and practice meditation. They must take full responsibility for the causes that led to their illness and find a new path for their life.

Tackling the root causes of Cancer is of utmost importance. Energetic healing practices can lead us back to the road to true and glowing health!

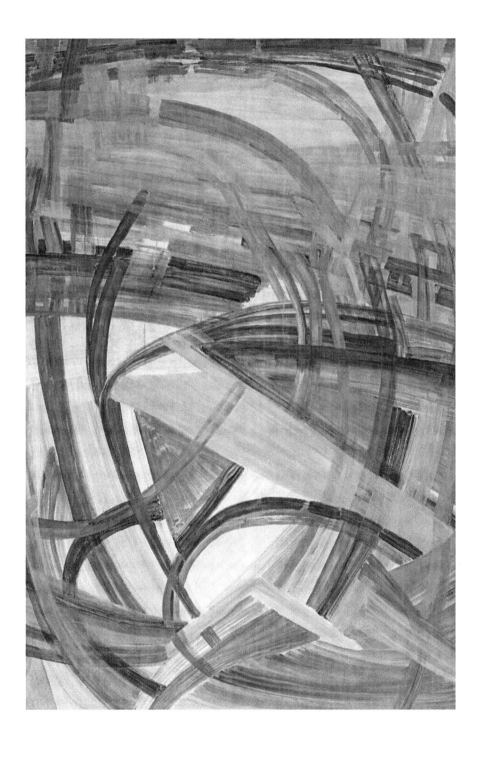

CHAPTER 20

Tackling Fear

LAUREL ANN REINHARDT, author of the book, *Healing Without Fear—How to Overcome Your Fear of Doctors, Hospitals, and the Health Care System and Find Your Way to True Healing*, had the difficult task of tackling her fear when she found a lump in her breast and felt the anxiety rising up within her. This scared her enough to go to a Medical doctor, though she was into alternative healing doing osteopathy, chiropractic, homeopathy and Asian medicine such as acupuncture, herbs, and Qigong for her health problems she had encountered in the past two decades.

The doctor seemed worried about the lump she presented and sent her for a mammogram. She says, "I didn't ask her about alternatives to having such a sensitive area of the body irradiated, or if the results of that procedure would make a difference to her or the surgeon, or if I could put off seeing a surgeon while I tried some other alternatives. I simply acceded to her recommendations out of fear."

Somehow she never received the postcard informing her that her mammogram was negative. Her next visit was to the surgeon who tried to aspirate the lump to find out if it was a cyst. Again she consented to this procedure out of fear. When it wouldn't aspirate, the surgeon recommended a lumpectomy. Her friend she had brought along reminded her to ask about options, including *options to surgery*. The surgeon grudgingly agreed she could take up to three months to try alternatives, but made no recommendations about what those alternatives would be.

Laurel Ann turned to her journal to help her find a path. She decided to trust her intuition. Her psyche had stressed joy and the need to consult alternative healers and her own self-healing abilities.

"Don't be afraid, fear makes disease stronger," her Vietnamese acupuncturist warned her. She got herbs from him and dietary advice from a nutritional counselor. "I began trusting myself, my dreams, and my own way of knowing again," she writes. Just as Kari had to face the fears of her family, her boyfriend Rob, and friends, Laurel Ann had to face the fears of her family, oncologists, and health care workers who warned her that she must do the medical treatment immediately. Despite this pressure, she decided to take personal responsibility for her fears and for her own healing.

Just as Shin had a client who had threatened to sue him, Laurel Ann also has an angry client in her psychology practice that had threatened her. She endured several weeks of sleepless nights from the resulting fear she experienced. She does not acknowledge this turmoil as a precipitating cause in her breast tumor, but she does write about it. Her entire book is about the topic of fear.

Fear, she points out, alerts us to the idea that something is wrong. Although it is often a first reaction to illness, she likened this emotion to a "friend ringing the doorbell." She suggested several methods of tackling this block to healing. The threat her client presented reminded her to "do onto others." She examined the way she treated people. Belly breathing, meditative walking, laughing, keeping a journal, recording dreams, and exercising are some of the antidotes she suggests to combat fear. "Fear is the preparation for movement," she points out. "A lot of power in America has been given to the Medical establishment, so our role as victims becomes ever more profound."

She decided not to become that victim. She did grief work, physically expressing and getting out her anger by hitting a pillow and scrubbing the bathroom floor until it shone, and grunting and screaming when she was alone. She then felt ready to express forgiveness. She then approached the people involved in this emotion. "Let them know how you approach your physical problem and how you would like them to respond to you and treat you,' she writes.

Since, as Ralph Waldo Emerson pointed out, "fear always springs from ignorance," her advice is to get as much information as you can about your disease. Response rates, she realized, only mean you are probably buying a matter of months. The toxicity of the treatment may not compensate for this short amount of time.

As her doctor felt she could have three months to try alternatives, she began to explore in what areas she could work.

I feel her deadline was an important part of her healing. Her dream-journal, exercising, nutrition (she gave up all greasy foods), herbs and group therapy did the trick. Within her deadline of three months, her body eradicated her tumor!

Laurel's program was quite similar to MOTEP. She took responsibility to heal herself, had a deadline, changed her diet, kept a journal, exercised, and practiced forgiveness and letting go of all repressed anger. We see she discovered how internal healing is far different from attacking a tumor. She followed her instincts, dreams, and alternative healers suggestions.

Why write an entire book about fear? I wondered. She gives exercises to overcome fear such as reporting, replacing, and releasing this emotion. She suggests discovering the inner smile, ritual and ceremony, prayer, meditation, visualization, using affirmations, and making sure that family and friends are only responsible for their **own** fears.

After thinking about it, I realized that she had an important point to make in Cancer. The Medical treatment is fear-based. The doctors upon finding a tumor become extremely fearful. They want to extract that tumor immediately and kill it. They want to use war weapons to wipe out Cancer cells, such as nuclear radiation used in deadly bombs and Chemotherapy used in biological warfare. Out of fear they want to drug, cut, poison, burn, and kill, kill, kill the dangerous and scary Cancer cells.

No matter how this treatment affects the patient, their goal is exterminate the Cancer with aggressive treatments at any and all costs! Even death! If you don't opt to submit to these "treatments" they are full of fear that they will get sued! They intimidate you by telling you that if you don't submit, the Cancer will spread! Cancer is fraught with fear. "We start living out the worst-case scenario, as though it were actually going to come true, as though it were already happening," she writes.

We might characterize this way of thinking as "negative visualization."

FEAR BASED PROPHYLACTIC MASTECTOMY

The ultimate in fear-based medicine is the prophylactic mastectomy. To me, this horrific procedure might be equated with removing your brain (lobotomy) if you have a family history of mental illness. After all, if you don't have a mind, you can't lose it!

A new study refutes the need to cut the breasts off of perfectly healthy women because they carry the mutated BRCA1 or BRCA2 genes. Usually women make their decision because of a combination of familial risk and "genetic counseling." Higher levels of *perceived* risk and worry imply a stronger intention for prophylactic mastectomy. But the fact is that a mutated gene only increases risk by eight percent. The other interesting fact is that mutated genes can become healthy tissue.

"Science Daily" reports "Cloning Embryos from Cancer Cells" in its June 4, 2003 issue. Nuclei removed from mouse brain tumor cells and transplanted into mouse eggs whose own nuclei have been removed, give rise to cloned embryos with *normal* tissues, even though the mutations causing the Cancer cells are still present! This finding was made at St. Jude's Children's Hospital and demonstrates that a Cancerous state can be reversed by reprogramming the genetic material underlying the Cancer. *The findings also indicate that genetic mutations alone are not always sufficient to cause a cell to become Cancerous. The environment of the gene mutation is more important than the gene itself.*

The fear that genetic counseling and family history of Cancer has led to the unnecessary mutilation and disfigurement of thousands of women based on the fiction (perceived danger) that gene mutations are the sole cause of a future Cancer. We now know better. Will this stop this hideous practice? Or will financial incentives win out? *Will fear win out*? It is our job to eliminate ignorance and put an end to the fear of future Cancer that drives us into unnecessary, destructive, mutilating "treatments" and procedures!

Carol, a woman I met on a house tour, told me that she had experienced Breast Cancer four years ago and had submitted to a double mastectomy with breast "reconstruction." On further questioning it turned out that she had merely had calcifications, a possible but not necessarily pre-Cancerous sign.

When I shook my head she said pointedly, "invasive calcifications." Calcifications do not "invade" or metastasize. This is usually a sign of stress, and I believe it can be fairly easily reversed on a de-stressing program such as MOTEP. "Why, that is like razing a house because there is dust on the floor!" I exclaimed.

She had submitted to an unnecessary surgery, an affront to her body, simply because of fear. If she had taken time to do some research into calcifications, she might have turned down this horrific amputation.

FEAR DRIVEN SCREENING MAMMOGRAMS

The fear of Breast Cancer has fueled the drive for screening mammograms. X-rays are a poor way to view breast tissue. Radiation is also carcinogenic! Scientists knew that for every one-to-two Cancers that they would find, they would actually cause three-to-five other ones! Yet a grant was given for mammography machines, and once again money won over health concerns. It is ironic that a test designed to detect Breast Cancer would actually *cause* it. But once again, the fear that "early detection" was the only way to "cure" Cancer, in some hazy form of thinking, won out. In 1997, the National Institute of Health was unable to reach consensus on screening mammograms for women forty-to-forty-nine. Mammograms had not proven their worth or accuracy in that age range. Finally, after a thorough study of the statistics, the committee decided to leave the decision to the doctor and his patient.

The acrimony and outcry from the breast community was intense! Thoroughly brain-washed, women cried out that it was unheard of that a woman should skip mammograms in their forties!

In the year 2000, Gotzsche and Olsen published their controversial paper questioning the value of mammographic screening in general. Six of eight studies done on mammography were found to be methodologically flawed. *There was no evidence that the screening decreased mortality in that age (forties) group.*

Psychological harm from false positives as well as over treatment of Ductal Carcinoma in Situ was found as reasons to discontinue mammography altogether. A statement appeared in "A Cancer Journal for Clinicians" in the June 12, 2003 editorial. "It appears that uniform and permanent agreement on screening for Breast Cancer with mammography may not be possible."

Alternatives such as MRI, thermography, dark-field Microscopy, and the AMASS blood test are never discussed when debating mammography. The AMAS blood test is nine-five percent accurate at finding Cancer anywhere in the body, is inexpensive, and can be done by any doctor. A small sample of blood is taken and sent to Oncolabs in Boston. (Telephone 1-800 9CA-Test).

Examining the blood taken from a pinprick by putting the drop of blood under a dark-field microscope is inexpensive, easy, accurate, and *non-carcinogenic*. Yet this test is ignored by a Medical Establishment enamored of high-tech machines and high-profit capability. This test shows how your blood looks throughout your body. If you have Cancer, your blood is inundated with white blood cells and the red blood cells are clotted together forming ropes. Looking at your blood will convince you that Cancer is not a local disease and that you must work on your entire system to get well.

In my own experience, I found mammography to be injurious, dangerous, and inaccurate. Kimberly's mammogram was negative, but a subsequent biopsy revealed she had Cancer. It's time we admitted that mammography is not the greatest idea for screening and looked at other safer, more accurate, and less expensive ways for diagnosis. Self breast exams and physical exams by experienced gynecologists should always be done to detect tumors. Often it is the woman herself who finds the lump, as in both Kimberly's and Kari's case.

CERVICAL CANCER REVERSED NATURALLY

Leila was diagnosed at age twenty-eight with Cervical Dysplasia, a serious first-stage cervical Cancerous condition involving the appearance of squamous cells. She heard me speak at the Goddess Gathering, a one-day seminar on women's issue, and was impressed that I embraced Cancer as a challenge. Though she found this "difficult to relate to" she knew she had met me for a reason. In April she went for her yearly checkup and her doctor found Cervical Cancer with a pap smear and a biopsy.

She decided to conquer her fears and try my MOTEP program to reverse her condition. Her doctor had recommended cryosurgery as her only option. This technique is old, dating back to the 1850's in England where it was used to treat advanced Cancers of the breast and cervix. A hollow stainless-steel vacuum-insulated probe is put inside the cervix that is chilled to minus three-hundred-and-twenty degrees Fahrenheit. The rate of cooling is important for tissue destruction. A hand-held ultrasound device is now used to monitor the extent of freezing. Once the tumor cells are frozen, the body will *theoretically* take care of the cells internally. Outside tumors form a scab.

Yes, I tell Leila, temporarily you can freeze the Cancer cells so that they stop moving and are even destroyed. But what happens when this area thaws? Will the Cancer cells once again grow? I believe they will unless you change the conditions of your life.

Leila demonstrated her courage by opting to try to change her life, rather than to submit to this temporary treatment "solution." When she first called me she was in a panic state. "My friends say that I am frantic," she admitted.

"If you are frantic then your cells are frantic too. That's why you have tested as having Cancer. Your cells are a mirror-reflection of your life-condition. *Your cells are you; you are your cells."*

At our first meeting she went over just some of her stresses. She had just broken up with her boyfriend of over four years. A " horrible roommate" left a nasty note when she had moved out. Her Mother had Lyme disease, an "incurable" affliction, and said she did not want to live! She had a conflicted relationship with her Mother when she first called me. Now she realized that in order to heal herself, she would have to change the relationship. She began talking to her mother every other day and looked forward to the calls. She considered moving up North to be nearer to her.

Her problems with her parents started early in life. Her father wasn't her real father, but she was conceived with a lover that left. Her mother then dated a lot of men, dragging her along as baggage. She recently did a conceptual art piece in which a friend got in a bag, which men dragged around. Only a hand showed out of the bag. She took a photograph of this strange, poignant scenario.

Leila was also bored with her job. But starting the MOTEP program, she realized she would have to confront her lack of interest in her work and expand her horizons. She began to take classes in Journalism, Photography and Criminal Investigating. She is now even considering an alternative medicine a career!

She began walking for forty-five minutes and doing weight machines for upper-body work. She began the MOTEP diet, eliminating her insatiable appetite for sugar. She also eliminated coffee and chocolate that contain caffeine that destroys the repair mechanism of the cells. "Chocolate and coffee were my favorite foods!" she exclaimed.

"Your face is clearing up," I noticed.

She nodded vigorously. I had observed that her bad case of acne was smoothing; glowing pink skin was replacing the ugly markings of pimples.

She also began working with a trainer one day a week. Besides walking every morning, she tried to fit in an activity every evening. She drinks carrot juice every day and has added avocado, oatmeal, bran and lots of vegetables to her diet. She bought a vegan cookbook and tried polenta with vegetables and brown rice with tomato sauce for dinner. For dessert she made banana-tofu pudding. She lost ten pounds in a month-and-a-half and looked slim and youthful. She set a deadline of four months from her May launch on the MOTEP program. Another pap smear would be taken at her gynecologists on the fourth of September. However, she moved up her deadline to two-and-a-half months so that she could get up on the stage with me at the Cancer Control convention for our lecture and video.

Setting a deadline is part of the visualization exercises. She mentioned she had problems with visualization, so we did a white-light meditation. We visualize a white light coming out of our eyes or third eye in the middle of our forehead. We accept this laser-like light as our healing source. Slowly and thoroughly we point this light at various areas of our body, one part at a time, to heal, cleanse and restore a feeling of peace within it. We spend about twenty minutes on this purifying, spiritual exercise.

Her final solution was to visualize a jar with white light, opening the jar, and releasing the light when she got to a different part of her body.

When we are done with our white-light visualization, we both feel refreshed and at peace. Leila, however admits the word "refrigerator" comes up and she can't ignore the problems in her home. She needs to fix the refrigerator. I advise her to practice this white-light exercise in the morning and evening until she can eliminate, for at least twenty minutes, her worries and concerns of her everyday life. Visualization is a time to transcend everyday worries. The body needs a peaceful environment in order to heal. *Establishing a peaceful internal environment is crucial for healing Cancer.*

Two-and-a-half months later she went back for a pap smear. Although Leila had told her doctor about my MOTEP program, her doctor said she did not believe in "that sort of thing," and had told her "Good-luck."

Leila had trouble retrieving her test results. "They didn't want to tell me my test was now normal," she explained. "She didn't want to hear that I completely changed my lifestyle and that had succeeded in turning my test results back to normal."

She was also enthusiastic about the "side effects" of my program which included feeling energized, not getting colds or flu, having a psyche she is comfortable with, and knowing she is an accomplished person. I also might add that she is now a beauty, having cleared up her complexion, gotten a better relationship, lost extra weight and become enthusiastic for her mission in life. When I had first talked to her, I had heard only complaints. Now on the stage, supporting me, she was radiant with health and vigor. "Most of all I am very thankful for these guidelines. I learned to listen to my body. Take Susan's plan and adopt it for yourself. I now listen to and trust my body. What is it trying to tell me? Everyone can adopt this plan and get healthy."

DR. LORRAINE DAY HEALED HER TUMOR NATURALLY

Dr. Lorraine Day has become famous for her dramatic story. Outspoken and energetic, Dr. Day was diagnosed with Breast Cancer eighteen years ago. As it was serious, diagnosed with a biopsy at Loma Linda University as an advanced Infiltrating Ductal Carcinoma, doctors told her, "You are going to die!"

"But they were wrong," Dr. Day exclaims joyfully.

She refused all their mutilating treatments including surgery, chemotherapy, and radiation. Instead she went on a ten-step all-natural program similar to my MOTEP program and healed herself in a focused, dedicated and whole-hearted way. Her program includes juicing thirty-six pounds of carrots a week, juicing leafy green vegetables, eating organic, vegetarian food, taking three-to-five mile walks, lots of rest, lots of clean, fresh water, deep breathing clean air, some sun, hours of prayer, and letting go of anger and resentment. The trigger points for her tumor, she believes, came directly from intense anger, the rage she felt toward her ex-husband. She had to find a way to release all that anger. Helping others became a mainstay in her life. Just like Laurel Ann, her first video deals with the emotion of fear: "Cancer Doesn't Scare Me Anymore."

Lorraine Day, M.D. was an internationally acclaimed Chief of Orthopedic Trauma Surgeon at San Francisco general hospital. She also worked for fifteen years as Vice-Chairman, Department of Orthopedics at University of California at San Francisco.

A beautiful, dynamic and vibrantly healthy blonde, Dr. Day saw thousands of Cancer patients die, not from their Cancer, but from the Medical treatment they were given at the hospital. An expert and author on AIDS (writing the book *AIDS: What the Government Isn't Telling You*), she spoke often at Lorraine Rosenthal's Cancer Control Convention on this topic. It was there that she inadvertently learned the truth about Cancer.

She listened to Charlotte Gerson talk about juicing and detoxification with fiber-rich fruits and vegetables. She heard recovered Cancer patients talking about exercise, prayer, and forgiveness. This helped her find the courage to heal her own Cancer with inexpensive, natural remedies. She states flatly that drugs *never* cure disease. "If you have just been diagnosed with Cancer or some other serious disease, do not be afraid," she cautions. "You have the power to rebuild your immune system and get well."

She has developed a small library of video and audio-tapes and has a web-site (DrDay.com). She travels the world lecturing on healing Cancer naturally. At the Cancer Convention she shows a slide of a grotesque tumor that looks like a grapefruit-size red rubber ball on her chest! It is a terrifying and shocking actual photo. This is the biggest, most horrific tumor I have ever viewed! It looks shockingly deep red and angry! She relates having severe emotional problems, fighting with her husband, and all the anger that consumed her.

Instead of being paralyzed with fear, however, she used the information she obtained at the Cancer Convention to turn her fear into energy and motivation.

Moving to the desert near Palm Springs, California, she began her healing journey. It took eighteen months of dedication: detoxifying, de-stressing, exercising, resting, and establishing a feeling of peace within herself by letting go of her toxic emotions before she slowly but surely was rid of her tumor and felt healthy and normal again.

Her videotapes explain why you don't need to fear Cancer. Instead of instilling fear, Cancer can be a motivator to find out the truth and learn to rebuild your immune system. "This is the only system that keeps you well. This is the only tool you have to get well from Cancer," she explains.

She points out how the American Cancer Society whose motto is "fight Cancer with a check-up and a check," makes four million dollars a year, most of it going into their own pockets. They like things just the way they are. They only sponsor research that utilizes the old, standard, outmoded treatments of surgery, chemotherapy, and radiation. They have no interest in mind-body medicine, how the body heals itself, or anything new for that matter! Their tight rein on the Cancer Industry insures that high income-streams over-ride the public's health. They, along with the pharmaceutical companies, control what the media tells us about our health. Thus we get a confusing and misleading message about Cancer.

"You can rebuild your immune system to conquer most

any disease. Don't be afraid," Dr. Lorraine Day advises. She is a most courageous, outspoken survivor. She learned how to conquer her fear and learn the truth about natural healing.

Laurel Ann, Kari, Leila, Cheryl, Orlan, Lorraine, Brandon, and many others are pioneers who did not let their fear of Cancer intimidate them into submitting to mutilating and poisoning "treatments". We will meet Deirdre and Shdema in upcoming chapters. All found the courage to heal themselves by changing their entire lifestyle. They found the gift of peace, health, and forgiveness. Helping others became a mission. They all impart this important message: **YOU CAN HEAL YOURSELF OF CANCER.**

CHAPTER 21

Shdema Goodman—
Healing Yourself from the Inside Out

SHDEMA GOODMAN BEGINS her seminar with the words "gratitude, celebration, and love." She urges you to visualize your desires to materialize. "Send me Love Blessings," she urges. "The more you bless, the more blessed you become. Chemicals of love and joy strengthen the immune system."

Shdema, whose spiritual name is Shivani, is like a goddess guide, conducting this Sunday's healing gathering dressed in a pale blue satin jacket and a white gauze skirt accented with pearls at her neck. She has long, glossy black hair that glows with good health. "Today we will embrace and transform negative energy and move on the path to a new level of growth," she explains.

Shdema has worked with billionaires and millionaires. She has found that it was not money that was important. Rather it was connecting to your essence. "The private jet is not the most important thing. Choose blessings. Whatever we have right now means we have what is good for us. Find your mission in life. Let go of your anger. It saps energy and stops growth," she observes wisely.

ACQUIRING HEALING WISDOM

How did this beautiful and forceful woman attain so much wisdom?

She was a practicing psychologist, she had her life "together," she was married and had a stable life. However after a vacation to Hawaii with her husband, Shdema realized she was afraid of him. She told him she would like a year off, a sabbatical from married life.

But this was not agreeable to him. He made it clear this would mean the end of their marriage. "What would happen to your hectic schedule as a psychologist in Boston?" he reminded her.

After some consideration, she decided she would like to try a life on her own. Her decision, not easily or hastily made, was to leave him and some time later to get a divorce.

SHDEMA CONFRONTS BREAST CANCER

A year after she had separated from him, in 1992, Shdema was diagnosed with Breast Cancer. The doctor advised a mastectomy followed by chemotherapy. Shdema dutifully followed the doctor's orders.

But this was, as so often happens, only a temporary solution. The problems she thought were going to be permanently solved the first time with surgery and drugs were still not solved with more surgery. One year later she was diagnosed with invasive, Stage Four Cancer that had spread everywhere. She was told to immediately check herself into the hospital or she would die.

Shdema is a staunch believer in following your intuition. She thought about this recommendation long and hard. You can see the confusion return to her face as she explains how she grappled with this tough decision. Yet she felt she had to make it herself. She is a leader rather than a follower. She was torn and tormented by the doctor's advice. Her struggle to make the best decision is evident as she explains the life-threatening situation that confronted her. Should she follow the doctor's orders? Her body twists and turns and a visible sweat breaks out on her brow as she recounts her wrenching, traumatic decision-making process and dilemma. The decision is one I have seen people go through when they opt for a natural path to healing. The Medical powers-that-be carry the weight of Establishment approval. They usually can intimidate the potential "Cancer patient" into submission.

Yet the Medical route had not worked twice before to stem the wild, out-of-control growth of her Cancer cells. That was the **fact** that confronted her. Still she was conflicted and confused.

Should she go the medical route that failed her before, or go on her own path of self-healing? Truly, the turmoil she experienced in attempting to come to any sane or rational choice was almost unbearable. The decision would have to be the right one! At this point she was facing down her own mortality.

Her strong feeling that came up was "If you go to the hospital, you will die in a few weeks. You won't be able to get in touch with your inner wisdom in that type of setting."

The Doctor called. "Are you ready to go?"

She told him "No".

Shdema began to cry as she tried to explain her decision

to him. She realized she "didn't have to do anything she didn't want to do."

Upset, the doctor warned Shdema that without aggressive medical treatments, she would not have long to live. She *must* come to the hospital.

"I'll think about it. I'll call you back. Good-bye." She hung up on him.

"We make doctors Gods," she explains. "But they don't have all the answers."

Shdema thought long and hard about what she should do. Slowly, a plan evolved in her frantic state of mind and her over-excited, jangled nerves. She decided to give herself three months to practice everything she had learned in psychology and from her spiritual masters. With this deadline and firm resolve in hand, she called the doctor back and courageously cancelled the hospital stay once and for all. She only felt tremendous relief. "Doubting doesn't work," she forcefully explains.

But the doctor was angry. He did not consider her decision a courageous one. "You're risking your life," he cried. "You're committing suicide."

Shdema realized that being sick had made her vulnerable. Yet she found the strength to stand up to him and make the decision that connected with her inner wisdom. Yet as firm as she was in her decision to go it alone, to be alone for three months and go on a self-healing journey, she found it difficult to convince her relatives. Her Aunt was indignant. "Who do you think you are not to listen to the doctors?" she exclaimed in horror.

But Shdema's decision had been made. She had a deadline and was firm in her belief that she could heal herself or at least begin to regain her health in the allotted time span.

She traveled back to Hawaii and went on her healing journey. She insists, as does Deirdre Morgan who has been a vegetarian for decades, that diet has nothing to do with it. (We will meet Deirdre in the next chapter). However, Shdema admits that she eats lots of organic fruits and vegetables. She relates how she drank lots of fresh juices. While both self-healers insist that healing power resides only in the mind and soul, both women follow a nutrient-rich diet. Both these women are spiritually advanced.

I advise going on a detox diet with carrot juice to further speed and enhance healing. One man healed himself on carrot juice alone after doctors closed him up after they found attempting to surgically cut out all the Cancer from his body would be futile. The mind is a powerful Cancer-healing weapon, but since the disease shows up physically in the body, why not treat the body too?

Shdema's healing exercises that we practiced in her Sunday seminar, involved relaxing the body and mind and then focusing on visualizing already being healed and well. "Give the painful area extra healing energy, she explains. "See yourself already well."

She did her relaxation and visualization exercises for one hour three times a day. She kept in mind her deadline of three months. "If I make it, I will devote my life to helping others," she vowed.

After three months the tumor had shrunk to half

its size. Encouraged, she continued **her** spiritual, meditative visualization exercises. The **tumor continued** to shrink.

Eleven months later, a doctor in Colorado confirmed that her tumor had disappeared. "A **mirac**le happened!" he exclaimed. "**Your Cancer is gone.**"

Off and on in her healing journey, Shdema was very sick. But her deep belief was that she could heal herself eventually. This is important. The body will automatically strive to heal itself. Shdema instinctively knew this basic foundation of healing.

When Shdema had regained her health, she decided to write about it. But she put off her book until six years later. Finally she decided to put her thoughts and healing program on paper. She decided *everyone can heal themselves*. She began to write *Nine Steps to Reverse Cancer without Chemotherapy, Radiation, or Dietary Changes*. This book is now available online and at her website: www.youheal.com.

She continues to do seminars. Her invitation to attend "Healing From the Inside Out—Opening the Door to the Love that Heals You" to be presented in Maui, Hawaii, is handed out. This seminar that focuses on *self-healing using only the mind*, promises more joy, more love, and more peace in your life. Her sessions are filled with gratitude, celebration, and love. These feelings bring a new radiance to the body. "The chemicals of joy strengthen the immune system," she notes. Love is an important healing energy. "Feel a ball of white love and bring that ball to your weak or painful area," she urges.

"What is your mission in life?" she asks our group.

For Joan, it was to "erase sickness and suffering from the planet." For Sally, it was to "dissolve obstacles within myself." For Jim, it was to "let go of arthritis and negative behaviors." For Julia, it was to "let go of illness, absolutely let go of it. When I'm not sure of what to do, I will let life come to me." For Allen, it was to live with his adopted family and fulfill his dream of becoming a musician. For me, it was to be able to teach people about Cancer so we can eliminate the idea that it is a "terminal disease." "If only they know how, people can self-heal their Cancer and experience no recurrences," I added.

Shdema nodded. It was eighteen years ago that she was first diagnosed with Breast Cancer. She says she learned not to dwell in an internal environment of negative feelings such as resentment, fear, pain, anger, jealousy, and hatred. "The right direction is passion, harmony, and a positive feedback system. Smell the flowers!" she exclaims. "Negative thoughts pull you away from your true nature. Move in the right direction, the positive direction," she urges.

"When you have negative energy around you, you can embrace and transform it," Shdema teaches. "Move on to a new level of growth and development instead of wallowing in depression," she urges. Her website also talks about and illustrates how our psyche—thought patterns, beliefs and attitudes are keys to our state of health. The real culprits are our toxic attitudes—unhappiness, scarcity, and negative thoughts are messages that we are not in alignment with our true nature. "Surgery and drugs only remove the symptoms, not the *cause* of disease which is psychological and spiritual.

"Unless the cause is healed, the disease will reappear," she notes.

Life threatening disease is often the unconscious solution when problems become overwhelming. Self-sabotaging attitudes are like poison to the body, disabling the body's immune system, ultimately creating disease.

"Seeing your symptoms as feedback is a way to see how to change your life. You can enlist the help of your imagination to heal. We need to identify our sabotaging thoughts so we can change them to healing decisions. Look inside at the decisions that have not served you and make decisions that can create a glorious life.

"Relax the body. When the body is relaxed, you will find love in your heart. Love is the most healing energy we have. When the body is peaceful, the natural healing mechanisms are triggered and the body can tune into its wisdom as how to heal itself."

Her twenty-minute exercise is divided into four parts: First tighten, then relax the muscles in your body one section at a time. Or, similar to hypnosis, you can count down from one-to-ten each beat getting more and more relaxed.

Secondly, you focus on stomach breathing, visualizing the healing power of the oxygen you inhale for another five minutes.

Thirdly, you change toxic thoughts to healthy ones.

Finally you connect to your inner healing abilities and strengthen and encourage them, giving extra energy to painful or problem areas.

This exercise takes about five minutes.

A physician from New York was diagnosed with Colon Cancer. Shdema taught him an ancient self-healing exercise, spending about five minutes. He was instructed to practice the exercise three times a day.

"I don't believe in this stuff," he said.

"You don't have to believe in it. It works anyway," she consoled him. (Author's note: The power of belief is very strong, and I don't condone this attitude.)

"But I'm going in for surgery next week," he argued.

"That's O.K." she reassured him. "Imagine that when the surgeons open you up, the tumor is gone."

"That 's impossible," he said laughing. "But I have nothing to lose doing it."

A week later he called to say that when the surgeons opened him up, to everyone's amazement, the tumor was gone.

Here is the five-minute exercise she taught him:

"Breathe love energy from the sun into your heart and solar plexus, located below your diaphragm. Feel the love as fire in your heart and direct that energy into your left leg. Allow the muscles to relax so that the energy penetrates the billions of cells in that area. Do the same with the other parts of your body, then send extra doses to the area you are healing.

Most importantly, see the area in your mind's eye as healed, perfect and shining with vibrant health at the same time that you are sending healing love energy to that area. Imagine the billions of cells blossoming into smiling flowers. According to quantum science, observers change what they observe with conscious or subconscious intention."

This exercise done three times a day can be supplemented with a one-minute version whenever you remember.

Shdema believes that when self-healing is practiced worldwide, we will have a more peaceful, healthy planet.

Her seven-day training program consists of nine topics:

1. Make a decision to be well. Decide to live in radiant health.

2. Heal your emotional pain. Release bad feelings and develop new healthy feelings.

3. Heal your toxic attitudes. Find the unhealthy attitudes that caused disease and make new healing decisions

4. Practice the daily healing routine. Relax deeply, self heal, affirm healing decisions, and consult the wise self within.

5. Call the Doctor within. Use wisdom within you to heal dis-ease and strengthen the immune system.

6. Use your doubt to create certainty. Put doubt in your doubts to create what you want.

7. Use spiritual energy to enhance your healing. Connect to your essence to access the love that heals.

8. Follow your heart's bliss and live with passion. Listen to the voice of your heart and create a healthy, fulfilling life.

9. Create a healing environment. Use the healing Circle to support your prevention and recovery.

Shdema has given us a spiritual and mental path for growth and wellness. Her methods work to relax and heal the body. She also shows us a path for creative growth and success in our work and relationships. She is a beautiful gift to the growing body of knowledge and leadership in the formerly negative world of Cancer and it's destructive, archaic treatments! She is living proof that the mental and spiritual components of healing Cancer are so strong that changing them into a positive, healing source is the one and only tool you need to heal Cancer, over-riding even diet and exercise.

On the MOTEP program, I include diet and exercise. Being the best you can be, the healthiest you can be, means getting into terrific shape. The body will respond to each encouragement from every direction. For complete healing and well-being, I strongly believe *every* aspect is important. Nutrition and lots of oxygen from exercise will support your spiritual and mental well-being as well as heal your body. Cancer cells cannot live in a highly oxygenated environment. Vitamins from fresh fruits and vegetables and their juice will aid your body in repair of damaged cells. Healing troubled relationships is of the *utmost* importance.

Shdema shows us, however, that even practicing using only the mind one can heal. It's truly miraculous. Even a one-method mind-program, if done with extreme focus, can work extremely well.

But why not have a great body too? Cancer is still a physical disease, even if it begins with an emotional and mental source. My conclusion? Do everything! The life you save may be your own!

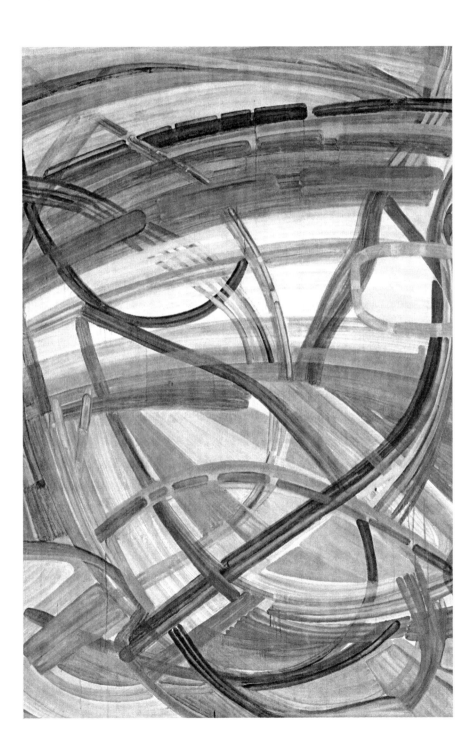

CHAPTER 22

Deirdre Morgan—Self-Healer and Sage

DEIRDRE MORGAN IS a wise and sophisticated world traveler. I met her when I was writing my first book on Breast Cancer. It was wonderfully fortuitous that I had randomly met another self-healer!

A vivacious, elegant woman, Deirdre had gone to her gynecologist at age forty-two for her regular annual check-up only to be shocked with the finding of a tumor in her breast. The doctor was firm that this was something not to be ignored and ordered a mammogram.

"At the time, I was too busy to stop or interrupt my schedule," she told me, her hands waving in the air. "I was a designer of maternity clothes and a trip to Saks Fifth Avenue in New York could not be postponed."

She did, however, get a mammogram, which proved the doctor correct in his alarm. The lump looked seriously threatening. The doctor called and ordered Deirdre to see a surgeon.

However, her trip lengthened when her mother, who lived in the East, was diagnosed with Gall-bladder Cancer and became very ill. "I felt an obligation to stay a month and take care of her. Deirdre's eyes got very wide as she exclaimed,

"My doctor was frantic and called everyday. He told me to get back and see a surgeon **NOW!**"

Her reply shocked him. "I do self-healing," she explained.

DEIRDRE'S SELF-HEALING PROGRAM

While taking care of her Mother on Cape Cod, Deirdre implemented her self-healing program. This is how she describes it.

"Every morning after awakening I would stay in bed and do visualization for twenty or thirty minutes. First I would focus on the third eye, the eye in the middle of my forehead, and think about and "see" a white light emanating from this eye. I would pull down this white light, letting it go throughout my body and circle it through my breast until I attained a peaceful, clean state."

She performed this white light spiritual cleansing only once a day. Along with this spiritual exercise, Deirdre supplemented her normally vegetarian diet by eliminating all caffeine and taking more Vitamin A and E. "I took about three Vitamin A pills a day."

Although Deirdre feels the vitamins strengthened her, the healing wasn't about any external substances. She feels that healing is an entirely internal process. "Find a wavelength and work with it. Accept it as a healing source." Then she quietly added, "There is a lot of motivation in Breast Cancer. I had to get rid of it.

"We need faith and trust in our own abilities to heal," she continued. "If we were really evolved enough, if we really believed, we would be able to use our spiritual strength to cure ourselves of anything. "We put "healing power" in a bottle. But what we really must do is empower ourselves. Get us to be true to ourselves and believe we can self-heal. The power to heal our own bodies lies within ourselves."

PROOF THAT HEALING POWER RESIDES WITHIN

Deirdre returned a month later, having gotten her mother through her catastrophe successfully. The next day her doctor set up an appointment with the surgeon.

After looking at the problem X-rays, the surgeon began the breast exam. He performed the manual procedure once, got a puzzled look on his face, and went back to review the X-rays. After three attempts to find a lump, he gave in. "X-rays don't lie," he said. "But you have nothing. I don't know what you did, but whatever it was, I suggest you keep it up."

That was twenty-five years ago. Deirdre is still wonderfully healthy with no recurrences. She feels there is a definite trigger mechanism. "You do it to yourself," she states. "Physical symptoms are easier to treat than the source of Cancer. However treating the physical symptoms won't always work. The mental and emotional core has to be dealt with. Otherwise, despite any physical treatment, the Cancer may spread.

DEIDRE'S THOUGHTS ON HEALING

Deirdre joyfully agreed to share her wisdom when I asked her to write about healing.

"When Susan first asked me to write about my bout with Cancer for her new book, I was very pleased. And then, after mulling it over, the reservations set in. Cancer is a highly personal experience. I will share what I feel is valuable and hope that it helps you.

"After getting the pronouncement from the doctor that I was tumor free, I skipped down the steps. I think we must all know that feeling of light-heartedness and joy mingled by tears of relief and gratitude. I bought flowers and lit candles that night. I put on Debussy and thoroughly loved myself. Meditation was easy that night except I didn't feel like sitting still. The next day, I bought myself a very expensive present. It was a bright new day and time to celebrate.

"And that is the first lesson I learned with Cancer: to acknowledge and celebrate myself. This had not been in my vocabulary prior to the scare. I had learned to organize my life around other people. My priority was meeting their needs and making them happy. I had bought into the role of 'Can-do-it-all-Superwoman, caregiver, provider, pretty Miss Perfect.' But Cancer was a wake-up call that made me realize that I had to take time for myself. I had to allot the time to heal from my own self-neglect.

"If you're like me, over fifty, perhaps you did the same things I did. I married young and had three sons right away. My husband traveled a good deal of time with his business. As a result, I submerged myself into the diaper and TV rut. I couldn't find babysitters, so my time off was very restricted.

"We moved to California and our marriage hit the rocks. Then came a vicious divorce—am I being redundant? What divorce is nice? I was out on my own then to make my own way, my own money. I was very frightened. My real learning began with having to believe in the power of the Self. Marriage had provided an illusion of a safe harbor.

"I actually had been working. I had employment as a corporate psychic and was teaching Yoga. I loved every minute of it. I'd also been running a natural ice cream shop in one of the beach towns close to where we lived. I owned the shop; however, it got sold in the divorce. Then I lost my job as a corporate psychic. I needed work in a hurry and jumped into the garment business.

"That makes little sense in retrospect. But I always had a great love of pregnant women. I think they are the most important people on the planet because they are creating life, the ultimate art form. And I thought most of the dress options back then were pretty bad and cutesy.

"So I plunged in, getting lost in eighteen hours of work, seven days a week. I know this is what starting a business demands. However, I was suppressing a boatload of grief, anger, and resentment towards the world. All these emotions I ultimately recognized as what I was feeling towards myself, for not speaking up, for not meeting my needs, and trying to be so wonderful for everyone else.

"I was about to find out that I hadn't made a healthy choice. As I was preparing for presentation of my line to Saks Fifth Avenue, I was diagnosed with Breast Cancer. To put it simply, my lack of self-respect and love had caught up with me!

"However, I think I was lucky. I'd come from a long line of women who had taught me that illness comes from one's mental/emotional state of being. Thoughts and feelings have a direct impact on our health. Even medical books state that up to eighty percent of illness is the result of stress and strain."

DOES STRESS CAUSE BREAST CANCER?

A study published on WebMD (Oct. 4, 2003), "Does Stress Cause Breast Cancer? Swedish study suggests that chilling out could lower Breast Cancer risk."

The study of fourteen hundred Swedish women started in late 1960, found that stress doubled a woman's risk of developing Breast Cancer. Women were asked if they experienced a feeling of stress for a month or more such as tension, fear, anxiety, sleep disturbances, or turmoil related to family or work problems. Women answering "yes" had twice the risk of Breast Cancer as women who managed to stay cool, calm and collected. This two-fold risk held up even when they looked into other risk factors such as family history of Cancer, alcohol use, body weight, smoking, age of menstruation, child-bearing and menopause.

CREATING HEALTH

Deirdre feels fervently that we are co-creators and participants in all the experiences of our lives including illness, except for congenital conditions. This includes the good, the bad, and the beautiful

"Life doesn't just happen. We are not helpless. The part of us that is God-like, that creative spark or force in each of is easily forgotten. The part that transcends the physical knows it is self-sufficient, self-contained and powerful, yet is fragile, easily discarded or scared out of us. That is what I knew I had to tap into again and form a strong and lasting bond. For I believed that we are all much more than our physical form. It was up to me to connect with the Light and to heal.

"Taking care of myself and meeting my needs has empowered me to give that much more of myself to others and to life. I'm having a dynamic life, teaching and guiding people. I love doing readings, working with people's core beliefs, which are hampering them from living their potential and creating their dream life.

From the great Within to the Great Without, I send love and light to you all."

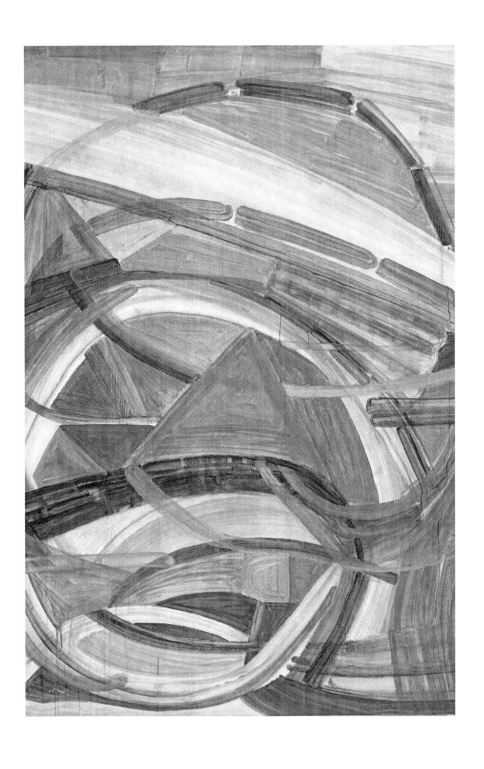

CHAPTER 23

Time to Heal

HEALING THE BODY takes time. The women and men I spoke to and interviewed made the conscious decision to take time off from their work and often frenetic lives to heal. They devoted their time to their health until they got well enough to gradually resume their lives. They assessed and took stock of the conditions under which they lived and worked. They spotted the problems inherent in their lives and instituted the changes necessary for good health to return. All the people I included in this book had the capacity to change and to grow. All of them took the time off to heal. Healing took all their energy. They took the time, willing to give any amount necessary to focus on getting well.

Cancer often takes years to develop. Under the impact of severe stress, depression and/or exposure to toxic and carcinogenic substances, the heroic defense mechanisms of the body will stave off collapse and degeneration for years before finally breaking down. When it does break down and a tumor forms or malignant cells start showing up, this is a message from the body that it needs time to heal.

TOO BUSY TO GET WELL

Melinda, a film producer, was diagnosed with Breast Cancer. She went to an Alternative practitioner, read many books, and began a supplement program. She called me about my Breast Cancer book, telling me it was so valuable to her that she often carried it around with her for inspiration. "The Doctor told me I had to submit to surgery," she said. "But I decided to do nothing."

After I hung up the phone with this vibrant, creative woman, only in her forties, it occurred to me that she had completely misinterpreted my book she had so praised. The MOTEP program certainly is not about "doing nothing." The program entails a lot of core healing work: doing the exercise, juicing, preparing the special diet, learning visualization and practicing it daily, applying topical, natural treatments, changing troubled relationships, eliminating stressful situations, going into group therapy, and reevaluating your whole life. Most of all, rest and sleep, *a lot of it*, are required to heal Cancer.

To get well from Cancer, a complex disease, takes a tremendous amount of time, work, and determination. It's about dedicating your time to your health until you get well. "Going to work" takes on new meaning. **Regaining your health becomes your new job.** This takes courage, self-reflection, dedication and spiritual strength. Other activities such as work must be sidelined or confined to part-time activity until at least a foothold on health is achieved. After all, adding years to your life is worth putting aside a few months to heal, isn't it?

About a month later, I once again heard from Melinda when she e-mailed me over the Internet. She had continued her high-pressured life-style, frantically pushing her documentary at various film-festivals she flew to, continuing the extreme stress that had most likely contributed to the breaking down of her health in the first place. Melinda wrote me she finally had gotten around to having the infected molar removed by the dentist that had been bothering her for some time. Meanwhile, her immune system, being further compromised by the tooth problem and unrelenting stress, had allowed bone metastasis. Oncologists wanted to do another core biopsy to determine the hormone involvement in order to find what drug to use: Tamoxifen or Herceptin. What did I think?

Dear Melinda,

Ironically, all the Anti-Cancer drugs are carcinogenic. Why do you need another biopsy? They already know you have Cancer. Hormones are a moot question now. The real issue is that you need to get well!

If I were you, I would STOP everything. Concentrate on healing. Stop the film festivals, all the stress, all the work, all the worry. Rest, sleep, exercise, do the juicing, practice visualization, chant and pray. You need to relax and let your body heal. **Do MOTEP full time**. You need to let your body heal and to support its efforts in that direction full-time!

Go to bed tonight and sleep twelve hours straight. Then get up and do the juicing and visualization. Next, go to the gym and exercise, sauna, and shower. Do weights, machines and sit-ups on the slant board. Be sure to deep breathe while working out. Next, swim if you like the water. I do half an hour of weights and machines followed by fifty minutes of swimming, taking a sauna in between. You can combine the sauna and the exercise with visualization for more powerful results. Spend a couple of hours. I do this three-to-five days a week. When I was healing from Cancer, I went five days a week.

Then go home and rest. Make a few phone calls if you need to, but your business needs to be put on temporary hold or on a very part-time basis until you get well. **You are fighting for your life**! I know it's hard to give up your film work and your hectic schedule, but it's better for now to give it up, at least temporarily, than to give up your life. You may have years ahead of you to devote to film But if you don't take the time off to devote yourself to getting well, your body will not have the energy or ability to save your life. Your body is warning you. I hope you heed it.

Best Wishes,

Susan

PURITAN WORK ETHIC

With our Puritan Work Ethic, it is often looked favorably upon going right back to work after grueling Cancer treatment such as chemotherapy or radiation, both of which are extremely carcinogenic, leading to fatigue. Then when the Cancer returns or metastasizes, why is this a surprise? Cancer treatment, as practiced today, only sets the immune system back further. The body needs even more time to heal than it would healing Alternatively, as both chemotherapy and radiation treatments destroy white blood cells needed desperately for healing.

Alternative healing demands focus and commitment. You are painstakingly looking at your life as you lived it in the last few years before being diagnosed with Cancer. You pinpoint the stressors, causes of depression, and lifestyle habits that strained your immunity to the brink of overload. You find a way to let go of anger and practice forgiveness with others. You reevaluate your life to find reasons to live and to get well. Then you initiate your healing schedule.

Armed with reasons to live and a full healing program, you encourage and energize your immune and healing systems to go into a high-gear healing mode. This initiates the healing processes.

Your own bodily "security guards" were laid off. You fired them when the distresses in your life overwhelmed you, you were careless about your health habits, or they got overloaded with toxins so they couldn't do their job properly. You must take the time to rehire them, to convince them that your life is worth saving and give them the ammunition needed to revitalize your bodily systems.

These guardians of your health will work for you again when you give them the time and pay them properly in care and attention. They don't ask for money. The body heals itself for free! They are totally efficient and effective. Once you convince them, by changing your lifestyle back to a healthy one and/or doing the emotional work and strengthening the will to live, that you are serious about getting well, they will take orders from you. They will do their job steadfastly and efficiently. In a short amount of time you will begin to notice results. My first "clinical trial," Belinda, reversed her problem mammogram back to normal in only ten days. That's how fast the body can respond when you make the decision to heal.

A PSYCHOLOGIST TAKES TIME OFF TO GET WELL

Dr. Norton Wyner is a robust seventy-seven year old Brentwood Psychologist I met recently. In his forties, he had been diagnosed with terminal Colon Cancer. He was told to have surgery immediately. He submitted to this surgery, losing eighteen feet of his transverse colon and had a bag for his waste products inserted. This did not make him happy. He instinctively knew this wasn't the answer to his problem and demanded that they do another ten-hour operation to reconnect his colon so he would not have to change a bag! He was then "given" three-to-six months to live.

To tackle the problem himself, Norton decided to take his life back. He planned a trip to the Adirondacks. In the forest, he rented a cabin and began what he calls self-hypnosis, putting himself into a trance-state in which he visualized his T-cells attacking and destroying his Cancer. He did this sitting down, lying down and while walking in the woods. "I was determined to get every last Cancer cell," he told me adamantly. "I knew I could do for myself what I taught my patients."

A Veteran, he had been injured and had to wear a corset brace. "I sat all day smoking three packs of cigarettes a day as I saw patients. Some days they couldn't see me because of all the smoke."

Norton decided to quit smoking. He also gave up alcohol that he drank throughout the day. "I'd have wine for lunch, a high-ball or Martini at dinner, and an after-dinner cordial. I also ate too much meat. I had a hamburger for lunch and a steak for dinner. I decided to become a Vegan and subsisted on vegetables, fruits, and whole grains for the next ten years."

In the Adirondacks, Norton also allowed himself to sleep and rest. Slowly he recovered his health in the brisk mountain air. With his new diet and without his addictions to cigarettes and alcohol, he knew in his heart that he had recovered his health and could return home to his family. He had taken a hiatus from family life, job stress, and abusive addictions and given his body the time and mental ammunition to heal.

He went to the Doctor who had give him a six-month prognosis at most. But the Doctor could not find any Cancer Cells in Dr. Wyner's body. "It's a miracle!" the Doctor exclaimed.

But Dr. Wyner knew he had helped create that miracle. He had dedicated his mind, body, and time to his own five-month trance-healing program. He changed his entire life to a health-oriented lifestyle and got well. It's been well over thirty-five years since his ordeal with no recurrence.

"I rarely work with Cancer patients because they are too distraught to be able to focus," he stated.

"I work with people who have addictions, using hypnosis and mental focus." He does work with Breast Cancer patients who are toxic from Chemotherapy. "We need to get those toxins out," he told me.

In a new research study, "Sleep affects Cancer," David Spiegel M.D. and Sandra Septon, M.D. found that poor sleep alters hormones that influence Cancer cells. Cortisol levels peak at dawn and decline throughout the day. This hormone helps regulate the immune system.

Melatonin is produced by the brain during sleep and may have antioxidant properties. It lowers estrogen production from the ovaries. Lack of sleep may inhibit Melatonin production. Night shift workers produce less Melatonin and their rate of Breast Cancer is higher. Researchers feel that hormonal patterns are affected by sleep and can predict Cancer progression. They feel that patients must allow themselves to get a good night's sleep and not worry about fulfilling obligations.[1]

Cancer TAKES TIME TO HEAL

In conclusion, healing Cancer takes time along with the implementation of a comprehensive natural healing program like MOTEP. Some people take trips to Texas, Mexico, the Adirondacks or Hawaii in order to heal. Others stayed home. **The body heals itself wherever you are.**

Some people need to get away from their everyday life and stresses, or opt for finding help in implementing a natural healing program, or just need to retreat to a place to be alone. My own solution was to turn my everyday environment into a healing center right at home.

Recently, I took a trip to Texas. I had been under unrelenting stress and problems. Rebuilding my studio wall just beating the rain by one day, having my truck break down in the middle lane of the freeway, having my art dealer cancel

---

1 "Brain, Behavior, and Immunity" October, 2003

a show of my work I had counted on, and banging the heavy studio garage door on my foot, all accompanied by financial stress because I could not sell my art in my damaged studio, I needed a break. I found a nice motel, went to bed, and slept for twelve hours!

Cancer FREE FOR EIGHTEEN YEARS

I was diagnosed with Breast and Uterine Cancer in December 1990. I have been well for eighteen years with no recurrence after healing myself. I celebrated by giving a talk on Breast Cancer at a new Chinatown branch of the Los Angeles Library where I was given a translator. Helping others is now a regular part of my life. I changed from being a self-centered Artist, only caring about me, myself, and I, to finding great joy in encouraging others to get well. **No one has to die of Cancer**. I firmly believe this now.

One of the principal things I learned about healing Cancer is to give the body plenty of rest and time to repair and restore itself. I've learned the importance of sleep. Now with even the greatest stresses, I've remained healthy.

All the people I interviewed who took the natural route to healing Cancer took the time to examine their life and stressors. They then took the time to go on an active healing program, devoting many hours each day to their routines. They decided changing their life was the most important part of their healing. They focused their time on getting well.

Whatever time they took will be made up in the future by extra years, many more years of healthy living. Take the time to regain and maintain your health. It's your most precious gift!

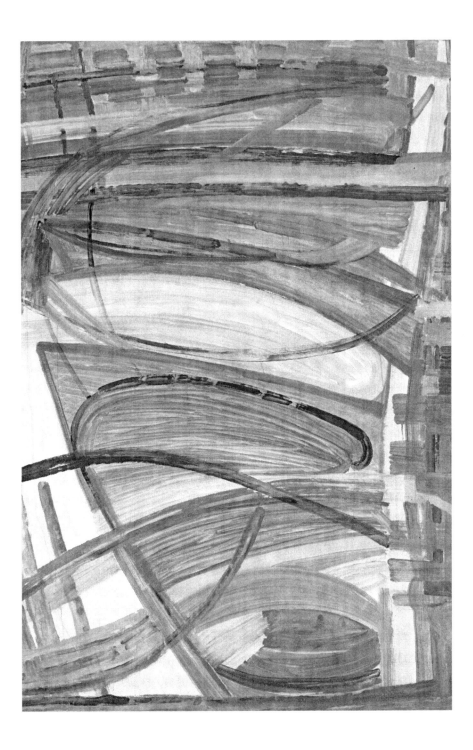

CHAPTER 24

Laugh Yourself Well—
Build Health with Creativity and Joy

GREAT COMEDIANS HAVE played a role throughout the history of mankind because they make us feel better. Laughter releases endorphins, nature's way of getting us high, feeling no pain, forgetting our problems, releasing stress, and making us well.

Fortunately, I met one of them. I didn't know at the time that Steve Martin would help me get through my healing from Breast and Uterine Cancers through his great sense of humor. But he did.

Was his movie "L.A.Story" possibly inspired by our connection? We'll never know for sure, however, my suspicion is that it was. It was at the premier I attended where I connected with him once more after meeting him in 1988. In the theater, I laughed and howled non-stop. How can you stop from laughing when Steve gets into his car to drive two houses down in a row of tract houses?

The funny thing is, I began to feel better. This was during a crucial healing period of my MOTEP program. I believe Steve helped me to get well.

I now believe he helped save my life.

Norman Cousins discovered this principal when he was diagnosed with a life-threatening disease, Ankylosing Spondylitis, a degenerative condition of the connective tissue of the spine. After a short time in the hospital, he made the decision to take charge of his illness. He didn't much like the sterile environment of the hospital, so he checked himself out of that uninspiring environment. Instead he got himself a nice hotel room and a pile of comedy videotapes and literally laughed himself well! Watching a Marx Brothers comedy film, he reported was worth two hours of pain relief! He subsequently wrote his timeless book, the 1979 best seller, *Anatomy of an Illness.*

He not only found out about laughter. He found out about inspiration, both from the environment and his spirit in creating health.

Endorphins released from laughter are hormones of pleasure and healing. They are very closely connected to our white blood cells, our healing apparatus. When we have a good time, lots of fun and laughter, we experience these healing hormones within. Natural killer cells are also revitalized when we laugh. Invigorated they can go about their job of destroying Cancer cells.

Many comedians live to a ripe old age. George Burns didn't go to heaven to find his Gracie until he was one hundred years old. "You drink, smoke, and carouse! What does your doctor say about that?" he was asked. "I don't know," George replied. "He's dead."

As a pubescent teenager, one of my favorite TV shows was "You Bet Your Life," starring Groucho Marx. Grocho was one of the Marx Brothers whose videos helped Norman Cousins reclaim his health.

The mustached comedian was the ultimate glib one-liner comeback guy who could flatten most any contestant unless they were super-sharp as one old lady he had on his show.

Groucho: "And what were people wearing when you were a baby?"
Elderly Woman: "Diapers."

In another exchange with a male guest, Grocho managed to get his point across.

Man: "I lived with cannibals in the jungle."
Groucho: "You're lucky you didn't go to pot."

Despite hard-scrabble early years in Vaudeville playing in cheap theatrical houses for peanuts followed by a long stretch of scrambling to make a living before he finally got his starring role on TV, Groucho lived a long life until age eight-seven, making others laugh with his irreverent humor and quick come-backs. He had three wives (not all at the same time), and wrote eight books. Of one of the volumes he quipped, "This book will have its usual phenomenal sales, and may even hit the one-hundred mark. Seventy-five copies of this masterpiece will be purchased by the author as birthday gifts for his immediate family, and the other twenty-five will be used to keep the window in the attic from falling down."

When he went on a war-tour for the soldiers, as Bob Hope was to do every war-year, his evaluation of the show's value to the troops was, "It's a distraction of inestimable value and cannot be measured in terms of just songs and jokes. When a show is advertised to appear, it is discussed for days before it arrives, and long after it is gone they still talk about it. From a curative standpoint, it contributes an element that no medicine can supply. Unfortunately he died in 1977. If he had lived two more years, he might have read Norman Cousin's book and found out how healing his "medicine of laughter" actually was!

Bob Hope who collected thousands of jokes for his personal files, and helped many squadrons of troops overseas by sharing them and making them laugh, also, like George Burns, lived to be one hundred. Despite having never been nominated for an Academy Award, he played Master of Ceremonies for the presentation many years in a row. He even made a joke about this disappointment. "In our house, we call this event Passover!" he laughed.

"I would have won the Academy Award," he added, "if it weren't for one thing—my pictures."

On his fourth hosting he joked, "This is my fourth visit presenting the awards. When it comes to an Oscar, I can dish it out but I just can't take it."

His longevity advice given in his nineties—"My secret for staying young is good food, plenty of rest, and a makeup man with a spray gun."

"My doctor says I've got everything going for me," he added. "Unfortunately he can't stop any of it from going."

The ability to laugh at one's foibles and disappointments instead of getting depressed and sulking seems to be one reason these wonderful comedians have such long lives.

Woody Allen's dialogue in his movie, "Manhattan," is revealing. His girl friend, played by Diane Keaton, breaks off her relationship with him and in the same breath announces that she is returning to her former lover—his best friend.

Allen responds passively while Keaton waits for a big fight to resolve the tension building between them.

"Why don't you get angry so we can have it out, so we can get it out in the open?" she insists.

"I don't get angry, O.K?" Allen replies. "I mean I have a tendency to internalize. That's one of the problems I have. I... I grow a tumor instead."

One of the big emotional contributors that may lead to a Cancer breakdown is repressed and silenced anger. Laughter helps release the tension caused by anger, resentment, jealousy and other negative emotions. Truth in humor.

Comedians are the world's therapists. They began, perhaps, by laughing at themselves to relieve tension and distract themselves from their own frustrations and turmoil. They found that laughing at themselves made others laugh. While Cancer is a "serious" disease and can be overwhelmingly threatening, the best antidote is to find something funny or ironic to laugh about. Try tensing up your body and laughing at the same time!

Madeleine shops at the organic market I go to. I noticed her one day because of her vibrantly beautiful facial complexion. Her skin was so luminous—clear and pink. She usually shops with her boyfriend, a handsome older man with white hair. I stopped her to ask if she would please reveal her secret as to having such beautiful skin. What did she use?

She began to laugh! "I'm eighty-eight," she informed me.

After she saw my astonished look, she laughed some more.

"Let me see your driver's license," I joked. "I don't believe you."

She admitted she completely stymied her doctor. "I've never seen anyone walk through the door who looked remotely like you at age eighty-eight!" she related, practically screaming with laughter. She gave no thought to what anyone in the market might think of her mini-riotous explosions of mirth, but just broke out into peals of pure joy.

She then revealed that she uses olive oil on her face every night, "just like Sophia Loren."

I began to implement her advice. Every night I rubbed my face and neck with extra-virgin olive oil before going to bed. This worked over the weeks to improve, moisturize and soften my skin that had been drying up with "age." After all, I was in my fifties!

But more importantly, I began to find more reasons to laugh. One reason is that a woman aged eighty-eight should indulge in having a boyfriend! "I don't want to marry again," she confided the next time I saw her in a low voice so not to disappoint him. "I was married for forty years!"

I looked at her again. She was wearing shorts and a loose cotton top. On her feet were socks and athletic shoes. I tried to remember if I had ever seen an "old" person wearing this type of sportswear, but came up blank. In my fifties I began shying away from shorts considering myself "too old" to wear them!

LAUGHTER IS THE FOUNTAIN OF YOUTH

The search for the Fountain of Youth has ended. The ability to stay young and to heal yourself of disease resides in the area of your laughter, your joy, your happiness, and your gratitude for life with all its splendid gifts. Healing happens when you create or enjoy the creativity of others—painting, drawing, singing, dancing, playing a musical instrument, going to a symphony, a ballet, a movie that is funny or uplifting, keeping a journal, writing a poem or book about your experiences, or expressing yourself in any creative activity.

You can tap into your healing powers when you create your own visualizations, think of a way to cheer up a friend *even though you're the one who is sick*, combine prayer with visualizations of the life you would like to create for yourself.

The best way to turn negativity and destructive thoughts around is to make a joke about yourself. When you see the irony or the ludicrous aspect of a situation, laughing about it can ease the anxiety quickly.

A visitor to my studio on our neighborhood Art tour asked me about my crayon drawings. Did I scrape through the layers of crayon to create a transparency where other layers showed through?"

"Yes," I answered. "I began using my fingernails. But after going through Menopause, I use a palette knife."

She laughed, looking down at her own meager fingernail growth.

Humor and creativity are entwined. Especially making up jokes about current difficulties and frustrations in your life takes creativity and a new absurdist view of your life. A tense, serious worrying eased into laughter. This creates an internal environment conducive to healing.

"Why is it that when I have an Artist as a patient they get well from Cancer, while other patients can't seem turn the disease around?" an Oncologist once asked me.

We Artists know how to access our creative ability and imagination that everyone has," I explained. "We know that illness gives us the opportunity to tune into that ability and *create* health. Healing is not a mechanical procedure. Drugs, radiation, and surgery are not creative. They do not challenge our creative healing abilities. In a sense, we artists see our bodies as malleable clay that we can mold, achieving what we envision. We know we have to do the work. We only have to use our energy, imagination, and power of transformation we know we have within us. When we are positive and willing to do the work of self-healing, we can create the results we envision. We've done it many times before with our creations. **Healing is really an Art**. All the scientific, high-tech equipment and cutting-edge technology can't reach our soul and our spirit where the true healing takes place."

The Oncologist only looked confused. My explanation had gone completely over his head. In his view the "standard" methods of treating Cancer did not involve any of the aforementioned things. To many oncologists, we are simply a robot with a tumor. Take the tumor out, destroy the Cancer cells with drugs and radiation—Voila! Now we are a robot without a tumor and exterminated Cancer cells. That means we are a healthy robot?

Cancer is not just a tumor. It's only one symptom. Yes, there are malignant cells. But the problem goes much deeper. The whole mind-body disease needs to be addressed. Root causes needs to be looked into. Lifestyles have to be worked upon. Real change has to take place. Slow and steady healing has to be gone through. Humor can help shine the way to true health.

HUMOR AS A RESCUE DEVICE

To regenerate an ill life condition, the spirit must be lifted. Humor restores our spirit. In turn, our health is restored. Smile when you look in the mirror, even if you feel like Hell. This sends your body a healing message. Rent some comedy videos or go to some comic movies. Find a friend with a sense of humor and talk to him or her. Make up or memorize some jokes. Tell these jokes to others. Everyone faces traumatic situations, depression, or overwhelming problems in their life at one time or another.

Even if you feel desperate about the doctor's prognosis, you can laugh at the idea that anyone without a genuine Crystal Ball can predict your future! **Prove him wrong**! Laughing in the face of threatening situations will diffuse the resulting upset. Only you can determine your fate. Take charge of your situation and turn it around.

WHAT IS THE KEY TO LONGEVITY?

Assessing longevity in a high-powered seminar the following topics were explored: caloric restriction, genetic engineering, antioxidant supplementation, hormone replacement, telomere growth and stem-cell therapy. All of these turned out to be futile in explaining why some people live to be over one hundred years old.

On a gerontology website, www.grg.org, the longest-lived person in the world ever recorded is described. A French woman, Madame Jeanne Calment, lived to be one hundred and twenty-six years old. She died in 1997. On the website she says her name in her French accent and sings several songs. Has this songbird found the secret to an astonishingly long life by using her voice?

A close contender for the title of oldest person in the world died recently at the age of one-hundred-and-fourteen years. She was a Japanese woman, Mitoyo Kawate. Kawate, who had four children, was a farmer in Hiroshima, working until she was one hundred years old. Kawate enjoyed custard cakes and liked to sing! Now we have two of the longest-lived people in the world who spent a great deal of their long lives singing! A photo of her alongside the article shows an ancient looking woman with a big smile on her face! Obviously, being old did not bother her a bit. She was too busy laughing and singing!

The list I would compile of what helps insure a long life would be much different than the "scientific" list above and would include: learning how to diffuse stress with laughter, counting your blessings, smiling whenever you look in the mirror, laughing with friends and relatives, helping others, sharing, volunteering, creating by painting, drawing, writing, acting, singing, composing songs, dancing, decorating, cooking new recipes, or creating new ones, exercising, loving others, and participating in joyful celebrations. Having a pet helps too. The black-and-white cat with a Lone Ranger mask and green eyes I recently rescued from the animal shelter, fills everyday with joy and love.

Whenever trouble looms, do the "lucky" exercise. Go over, one more time, how lucky you are and the advantages you have. Forgive everyone by laughing at your past feuds. What was silly about your fighting?

Humor creates hope for a better result the next time around. Humor saves and extends lives. Take a lesson from these long-lived people. Laugh and smile and sing your way to health and well-being. Bring healing into your everyday life with joy and creativity.

CHAPTER 25

The Cancer Personality—
Emotional Links to Your Health

A CONTROVERSIAL TOPIC, the Cancer Personality is a subject much argued about. One argument is judging your personality creates guilt and blame. Nevertheless, without "blaming the victim," we can learn much about how we can recover health and stay well by examining our emotions and how we do or do not express them. The Chinese believe that the emotions are *always* involved in Cancer. I believe they are right!

Lydia Temoshok, Ph.D. discovered over and over that her Melanoma patients had similar personalities and ways of not dealing with their emotions, mainly not being able to express anger. She wrote the book, *The Type C Connection— The Behavioral Links to Cancer and Your Health.* She found her Cancer patients to be always and, without exception, exceedingly *nice.*

Nice-guy behavior is directly associated with repression of one's darker emotions, she points out. She feels that helping Cancer patients to assert themselves is empowering and aids in healing. This helps them to regain the fighting spirit so important in Cancer recovery. Temoshek calls it grit, determination, and faith in one's own healing capacities.

In his book, *Spontaneous Healing*, Andrew Weil, M.D. talks about emotions and healing. "When I see patients whose lives seem out of balance, whose energy levels fluctuate wildly, who eat erratically and have unstable relationships, I usually recommend breathing exercises and meditation as methods to restore balance. But when I look at the role of emotions in facilitating spontaneous healing, it may be more useful to encourage sick people to cultivate passion." He found people with Cancer to be apathetic. He mentions falling in love or expressing anger as emotions that help healing. Two radically different approaches.

Actress Bonnie Hunt was an Oncological Nurse before she made the big decision to follow her dreams and become a movie star. Bonnie says her Cancer patients urged her on. "When they got Cancer," she observed, "they lost their fear." She points out another emotion that may be involved in Cancer before its actual diagnoses.

MY PERSONALITY

In looking at my own behavior, I found that I was a fairly typical Type C personality when I got Breast and Uterine Cancer. At the time, anger was the hardest emotion for me to express. People have commented that I am overly polite in many cases. I was really nice! (Sometimes, anyway.)

Many times this was only a façade covering up a tremendous amount of anger. I think I also had tremendous fear and a dark depression, having temporarily lost my passion! A man had left me that I thought I was madly in love with. I found creativity blocked because of this depression and tension about my future. The anger I felt when he married another woman was never expressed.

Even in the first grade, I was commended for being so quiet. I never made any trouble or got into any fights with anyone. But I was extremely good at being a victim and a scapegoat for other's anger and pranks. These days, I have to be on my guard not to return to that role. I have learned, finally, to stand up for myself!

The boy who sat behind me in the first grade was a rascal. The policeman's son, he knew how to get into trouble. For instance, my Mother bought me a beautiful velvet hat. He stole it and stuffed it down the toilet. My Mother bought me another one in a different color. It suffered a similar fate. Then I brought the first dollar I had ever saved to school. He stole it. The result was I got a beating at home from my Father because I took the risk of bringing my money to school. As a small child, I could not stand up for the unfairness of this beating. I was totally helpless.

I never blamed the boy who sat in back of me, and he probably never got punished. I always knew he did this to me, however, and I think he eventually turned to a life of adult crime. Why didn't I get angry with him? Probably because I was afraid of what he would do to me if I did express my outrage.

My father was an angry and violent man at times, taking his wrath out on my brother and me. I was severely punished with beatings for anything and everything, even when I did nothing wrong. This led to a fear of people and of standing up for myself in situations where I was insulted, mistreated, or taken advantage of. Because my father used me as a scapegoat for his frustrations and feelings of inadequacy, I became quite comfortable with that role and easily fell into it with others. I really love my father with all my heart, so I accepted that he must be "right." I thought I didn't deserve to be treated well.

This pattern continued until I gained confidence as a swimmer. My father was a championship swimmer in college, and early on taught me how to swim. He often went swimming with me as a child, which I loved. I also took the lessons offered at the local pool and moved up quickly to the advanced classes, synchronized swimming where we gave performances, and finally to lifesaving classes. It was there that I finally learned to be strong and to fight for my life.

During the first lifesaving class I took (and flunked), I helped save a little boy's life. He had dived off the diving board and failed to come back up. One of the guards dove in and pulled him to the surface. Others pulled him up out of the water to the pool's edge. On the concrete, I helped give the artificial respiration that brought him quickly back from his non-breathing, blue state. Although it only takes three minutes without oxygen to kill a person, because of our quick, informed rescue efforts, he survived.

However when it came to saving the instructor during the final test, I almost drowned. I just didn't have the energy, confidence, strength, or single-mindedness to fight back as hard as I possibly could. My parents took it well. Only being a sixteen-year-old skinny kid, they excused me. I had merely to lean on my victim story.

However the instructor wasn't satisfied. I guess he saw something within me that could become a success story. He didn't want me to remain in the victim role! He told me he was offering another class for the Boy Scouts and he wanted me to take it! I said I wasn't interested. I was too young to have much of an interest in boys, and I certainly had no interest in drowning!

But he kept after me.

Finally, one day he convinced me. He told me there would be one other girl in the class and she was handicapped, having had polio in her younger years. I visualized this poor girl having to deal with a class full of Boy Scouts, felt sorry for her, and agreed to take the class.

One day in our practicing, Ed jumped into the pool. He was the head lifeguard and big six-foot, two-hundred-twenty pound guy. However, I liked him and somehow I knew I could meet his challenge.

"Come get me, Susan," he taunted me.

I dove in. Where had the confidence suddenly come from? He knew me. I intuitively knew he believed I could win. He had supreme confidence in me. And he fought like a tiger. When I had successfully "saved" him, there were fingernail scratches all over his body.

After the poor handicapped, crippled girl (who proved to be quite strong) and I showed up all the Boy Scouts on the final test, making them all look insipid, Ed hired me to be the youngest lifeguard at the newly built indoor pool. I began earning money guarding and teaching children to swim, buying my parents Christmas gifts with my own funds. I bought a candy-apple green Ford that needed work and almost got stuck on the railroad tracks with a train coming at me and a carload of girlfriends. However, my newfound courage and confidence saved the day. I got the car started in the nick of time and backed off the tracks, only to look up and see the train in the exact spot! My new belief in myself, nurtured by

Ed the head lifeguard and my new job, had given me a confidence and sense of control I had never had before.

I had a new status. No longer was I just a wallflower, a shy quiet victim of my own insecurities. Now I was a fighter who succeeded in defending myself, fighting for my life, and rescuing others. I had a job that paid well, and I had respect. More than that, I had learned to stand up for myself, to fight for what I wanted, and a way to tap into the courage and confidence needed to overcome gigantic obstacles.

MEETING LIFE'S CHALLENGES

I found in life that I was challenged again and again. As an artist, I had three studio fires (though I never lost a painting in any of these fires due to fast-acting firemen), financial ups and downs, emotional turmoil due to many failed relationships, and health problems to conquer. However, Cancer was the biggest challenge I ever had to face. I had to learn to fight for my own life! This took the courage to take responsibility and the determination to turn my deteriorating condition back into health one step at a time.

A passive approach was not, by then, my style. This take –charge attitude and the ability to take action, to devise and follow my own MOTEP program, was, I believe, the greatest contribution in my getting well and staying well for eighteen years so far.

In the Medical literature I found that "passive patients fare the worst." My friend Kimberly had taken just this attitude toward her disease describing herself as a "Cancer Patient." She told me she was going to follow the "traditional" way of dealing with the disease and just "do what the doctor says."

Kimberly just wanted to lie there and take whatever treatments they prescribed. This made me angry. I knew, intuitively, that this would not pull her through. But what could I do? She only started asking me questions at the point where she foresaw her own death, when it really was too late. She was only thirty-eight when she died a most miserable, tortured death four years after she found the breast lump herself. I strongly believe she died from the brutally harmful Medical treatment she received.

When the Doctor had advised her to meditate, she tried but soon gave up. She preferred to let the treatments act to "kill the Cancer," she told me. Unfortunately, they also killed her.

Every year at Christmas time, the pain of losing this beloved friend is very great. She had delighted her friends with a lovely, warm Christmas party each year.

SINGING YOUR SONG

Lawrence LeShan, who wrote the marvelous book, *Cancer as a Turning Point*, found his Cancer patients had an inner frustration of long-standing because they weren't "singing their song." These people with Cancer had suppressed what they wanted to really do in their life, sacrificing themselves to others. When they discovered reasons to regain enthusiasm for their life, they frequently recovered their health.

He writes: "The person exists on many levels, all of which are equally real and important. Physical, psychological, and spiritual levels are one valid way of describing the person, and none of these can be reduced to any other. To move successfully toward health, all must be treated. All must be taken care of and gardened if health is to be maintained."

SARA REGAINS HER HEALTH

Sara, in her late forties, was a high-powered Public Relations agent. Actually, she disliked her work, but was reluctant to give up her success. Her marriage was "friendly" but devoid of passion. She had no children. She had abdominal pain that was diagnosed as Stomach Cancer with metastases. Chemotherapy was recommended without optimism. Her husband was told to expect a rapid decline and an end to her life within probably eighteen months.

She asked her husband for the truth. Sara then decided that the Medical Program was not promising enough to offset the side effects. She determined to design her own program from whatever sources were available and began to investigate Alternatives. She began with a Nutrition program despite her Doctor's objection that it was useless. She also began a sensory awareness class and began to study a meditation program that she instituted twice a day. She began psychotherapy with a therapist who concentrated on what was "right" about her, not what was wrong. She also looked at ways of being in which she could find the most joy, zest, and serenity. She began to explore what was "blocking" this in her life.

As a result of this search, she decided a large paycheck and prestige were not enough for spending forty of her best hours a week at a job she hated. She resigned and began a new career of life coaching, which she thoroughly enjoyed. She was now glad to get up in the morning and looked forward to going to work. Two evenings a week, she volunteered for a group that helped former convicts turn their life around. She also got her husband to change and grow with her by getting him into psychotherapy. They discovered they liked each other more, and their marriage that had gone stale began to improve.

The year after Sara started her new life program, her tumors regressed. Six years later, she was completely symptom free: X-rays showed no sign of Cancer. To mobilize her self-healing capabilities, she worked on her life on all levels. She took charge of her healing, making her life worth living thus strengthening her will to live. By redesigning her life, she redesigned her health.

PENNY FINDS HER PATH BACK TO HEALTH

Penny Brohn is a personality that fit the Type C pattern at the time she was diagnosed with Breast Cancer. She had a difficult childhood living with her lay preacher grandfather and infinitely judgmental mother. At age thirty-five, she was found to have a breast tumor. The year was 1979 and she had just gotten an acupuncturist certificate, returning from Hong Kong where she studied, to her home in England.

In the Orient she had lost her social connections during her studies and was depressed, confused and groundless. Her father had died unexpectedly while she was away. Her mother, feeling she could not live without him, followed him into death eight weeks later.

Penny had been married fifteen years by then and had three children. She found she had been unhappy for a long time. She predicted something really terrible was going to happen to her.

Her doctors scheduled Penny for an immediate mastectomy to be followed by chemotherapy and radiation. She refused. She had just spent months studying holistic medicine and found "she just couldn't do the surgery recommended." Penny did the research and "It looked to me that Breast Cancer statistics for conventional treatment were still not much better than they had been in 1908."

Her doctors were horrified that Penny would not submit to their treatments. She agreed only to a biopsy that proved longer and bloodier than expected when a large mass was discovered. It was malignant. Hurried preparations for surgery were made, but Penny balked. "I was done being a passive recipient that night. I would not be rolled over into taking this major step." This was a drastic personality change. Coming to pick her up, her husband wondered, "Where is the woman who is such a wimp, she'd say anything to please everybody? What happened to her? She was gone!"

She and her husband David flew to Bavaria to work with alternative doctor Joseph Issels. She stayed nine weeks to do the entire program. Homeopathy, naturopathy, and fever-inducing immunotherapy were parts of the program. She found the psychological part most essential, especially the part of having a hard time expressing anger to defend herself. "Not too good at that," she admitted. Penny decided to spend time each day stamping her feet and getting rid of repressed anger.

With a friend, she made a decision about a new direction for her life. "The Heck with it, whatever else happened, if I lived long enough, I was going to set up a center for people who have Cancer," she explained.

That was her *turning point*. Penny had been quite low, but now thinking of helping others, she was able to reenergize herself. She literally got up and began to plan.

A combination of relaxation, alternative treatments, and having a glorious new goal for her life, worked to help boost Penny's immune system. Her tumor melted away.

With a partner she opened a Cancer center in Bristol, England, in a former convent. Her program was improvised from her experiences in Germany, Chinese Healing methods, and body-mind-spirit emphasis. Her goal: "To unshackle patients from a self-fulfilling prophecy of death."

"If I could somehow show them that even one person in the whole wide world had managed to turn this thing around, it would give them hope. It seemed to me that nowhere in the hospital system was anybody getting the message that it might be possible to wrestle with terminal disease and succeed."

At her center, Penny taught relaxation, visualizations, nutritional counseling, and spiritual approaches. "Most important of all, we had group sessions where everybody sat around in a circle and talked."

Soon the center was featured on TV and they were inundated with patients. Prince Charles even lent his support.

Four years later after opening her center, Penny experienced a recurrence. Two lumps appeared in her breast, one infiltrated. She decided again to attempt to heal herself and she succeeded!

Now Penny is a two-time winner and best-selling author of a book, *The Cancer Prevention Book—A Complete Mind-Body Approach to Stopping Cancer Before it Starts,* written with Rosy Daniel, M.D. and Rachel Ellis.

What can we learn from these examples?

1. Medical prognosis is based solely on results from Medical treatment. No one can predict how long you will live. Defy the prognosis and set a goal as to when you will get well.

2. What is right for your personality? How can you build on your strengths to enrich your joy in life, your enthusiasm and desire to get up in the morning? What is blocking you from achieving a rich, rewarding life.

3. How can you better express your feelings? If you have taken the victim role for too long, how can you better stand up for your rights? How can you take a stand for your own personal happiness? **You deserve to be happy.**

4. If you are married but not happy, what can you do to change your relationship? Take action to change or end a bad marriage. Your body is telling you something. Listen to it.

5. Cancer does not have to be the end of your life. Explore the problems in your life and why your body has reached this "dead end." It may be just a temporary **STOP** sign.

6. Many Cancer Survivors, including me, describe Cancer as a "gift." Helping others was not in my program as a self-centered artist before my body was inundated with selfish Cancer cells that are users and destroyers. I learned my new mission

in life is to help others learn about how to get well from Cancer. I destroyed my selfish lifestyle. In doing so, I destroyed my Cancer cells.

7. You can get well from Cancer. By discovering the "causes" in your life and beginning a new life, new diet, new exercise schedule, meditating and praying, helping others and changing your life, you can retrieve your health and well-being.

8. The Cancer personality often has conflicts in relationships. Work on mending your relationship with others, make peace with your parents even if they are no longer with you, harmonize your relationship with your spouse or primary relationship and your children if you have them, your associates at work, and especially your relationship with yourself. When you are fighting and out-of-sync with your environment, your cells mirror this and become chaotic too. Establish a feeling of peace within your daily life and your cells will reflect that inner peace. Your cells are you. *You are your cells.*

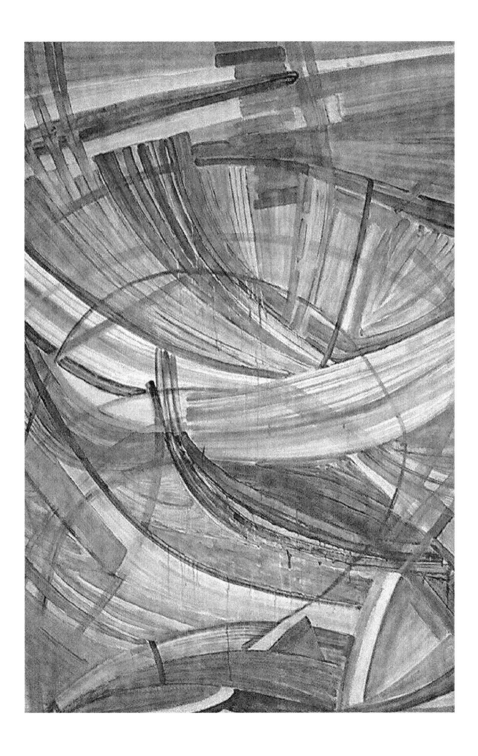

CHAPTER 26

The Trouble with Assumptions

THERE ARE MANY assumptions that go along with the disease of Cancer that need to be examined in depth and even dispelled. First and foremost is the generally accepted, depressing, downbeat idea that Cancer is a Terminal Disease.

The long line that forms each year to give testimonies at the Cancer Control Convention, people who used Alternative means of regaining their health, continually amazes me. These people are free of recurrences and actively do the work to stay healthy. They gave up smoking, high-fat diets, and learned about how to handle stress. They went through detoxification for their bodies. For their minds, hearts, and soul, they forgave people they had held grudges against, got counseling for their depression, and learned a positive approach to their lives. They incorporated exercise into their schedule. They found new ways to help others. They gained a new and profound appreciation for their lives. Often they tell me that Cancer was the best thing that ever happened to them! It gave them a new appreciation for living.

For too long we have assumed that a Cancer diagnosis means almost certain death. This death would be cruel, painful, torture! It just doesn't have to be that way. One must not develop a fatalistic attitude upon diagnosis, because this attitude actually facilitates a downhill course. Physicians need to reconsider giving out a prognosis of a certain number of months or years. The whole idea of prognosis is absurd and dangerous. No one, even a doctor in a spotless white coat, can predict your lifespan. No doctor, however informed and competent has a Crystal Ball!

TAKE TIME TO MAKE YOUR DECISIONS

The assumption that Cancer is an emergency situation that demands immediate treatment must also be challenged. According to Fran Visco, Chairman of the National Breast Cancer Coalition, people should do their research, reach out to other individuals who have had Cancer, and make their own decisions.

"There is time to do research after diagnosis, and there is a great deal of information out there," she states. "For instance, everyone gets chemotherapy, yet the majority of women with Breast Cancer do not respond to chemo."

DO DRUGS SOLVE THE PROBLEM?

There is another assumption that definitely needs to be questioned. Does everyone with Cancer need toxic drugs, or is there a better, more humane and healthier approach? In their one-sided view, the American Cancer Society has overlooked a natural vitamin, Vitamin B-17, or Laetrile, that the body can actually utilize to rid itself of Cancer cells and substituted dangerous and destructive drugs that they can sell at an exorbitant price. Current rates for treating Cancer with "standard" Chemotherapy can reach a half-million dollars! These toxic drugs destroy the immune system, gastrointestinal tract, and harm the heart, liver, and lungs, destroy fertility, and destroy bone tissue leading to osteoporosis. Even the brain is partially destroyed, currently acknowledged as "Chemo-brain syndrome." Secondary Cancers are often created from the loss of white blood cells; the immune system is destroyed by these toxic drugs. The death report often states that "patient died of *complications*" of Cancer or of Cancer treatment if they are honest.

IS RADIATION A THERAPY?

The assumption that radiation is a "therapy" must also be questioned. According to Wendy Silverberg, M.D. at the Department of Radiation and Cellular Oncology Department at the University of Chicago, one quarter of patients treated with adjuvant radiation develop Lymphodema, a swelling of the arm that can eventually paralyze it. Older patients are at the greatest risk, according to a retrospective study. Over-treatment of Cancer patients is currently being questioned, including the routine use of regional radiation. In its zeal to destroy Cancer cells with carcinogenic radiation, the medical establishment fails to think about the additional Cancers that may occur years down the line from these treatments. Cancer may appear twelve or more years later from the use of radiotherapy.

"Locoregional recurrence after surgery, chemotherapy, and radiation therapy for early Breast Cancer is common," according to a study in the medical journal "The Breast" (October 9,03). The recurrence shows up in skin of the chest wall where the breast used to be, surgical scar, axilla, ispsilateral breast tumor recurrence, infraclavicular lymph nodes, supraclavicular fossa lymph nodes and internal mammary lymph nodes.

"Due to the variation in sites of recurrence, time since initial diagnosis, and prior therapy, the exact prognosis and optimal management of these locoregional recurrences remain undefined."

Usually the approach mimics the treatment at time of initial presentation of Breast Cancer.

The assumption here is that the treatment given in the first place worked, but the Cancer returned. But what if it didn't work? The "recurrence" is only the same Cancer they did not know how to treat in the first place! But they could never admit their treatment was worthless. So instead they assume it did work and the Cancer merely "recurred." So what do they do now? Usually they give the same treatment that may have not worked in the first place!

So now we have it in plain language. No obfuscation with "scientific" sounding terms.

The hope is that the same treatment will work the second time around. But too often the Cancer returns with a vengeance, showing up in many more organs and areas of the body.

When this happens, instead of saying they give up, they state that treatment is now "palliative," a blanket term that translates to a treatment that won't produce any results and is completely ineffective!

The major assumption this treatment is based upon is that disease can be cut out of the body. After that, the disease can be poisoned and burned out. What other disease do they think they can cut out of the body? The flu, a cold, measles and mumps were never considered "candidates" for surgical intervention. Because Cancer often shows the symptoms of a tumor, surgeons assume that cutting this symptom out will cure the disease. This assumption is based on fairy-tale thinking. It's impossible to "get it all." ***Cancer is always a systemic disease.***

Cancer is a state of degeneration of the entire body, mind, and spirit, not just a tumor. ***The assumption that the tumor is the Cancer is a dangerous one.*** A patient whose tumor has been surgically removed may believe mistakenly that they are "cured" of Cancer.

VALERIE'S BRAIN TUMOR

Valerie, a beautiful woman in her thirties, developed a brain tumor slightly smaller than a golf ball, four years after being in a plane crash. The plane had to belly-land in a field after its wheels failed to lower. The seat belt she wore was powerless to hold her in her seat with the massive jolt the plane took upon landing with a gigantic ear-splitting thud. The tremendous force of the landing pushed Valerie to the plane's ceiling where she smacked her head with a shocking, violent thrust.

Valerie is a slim energetic mother of a seven-year-old son. I met her at a conference and liked her immediately. She is French and talks a mile-a-minute, enthusiasm for her goals in life is readily apparent. She is a weight-loss consultant, having victoriously lost one hundred pounds of her own.

When a brain tumor that formed in her skull two years after the plane accident proved to be malignant, Valerie was recommended for immediate surgery.

"I couldn't see my head being opened with a knife," she shuddered. I said, "NO."

Instead Valerie took up jogging, which she intuitively felt she needed, although her doctor advised "no exercise." She ate only fresh, whole organic foods and had a barley and mushroom recipe to share. (I found barley to be one of the best detoxifiers in my MOTEP diet).

Valerie also gave up her "enemy" list. She had formerly compartmentalized anyone who disagreed with her viewpoint as an "enemy." The resulting animosity and resentment combined to create a hostile, tense state, which she thought might have contributed to her tumor.

In six months of her intuitively formed health program that was amazingly congruent with my MOTEP program, her tumor had miraculously disappeared. Her doctor was astounded when he gave her a clean bill of health. He had never seen anyone heal a brain tumor naturally, without a lot of medical intervention.

Doctors assume this is "spontaneous remission" and give credit only to some mysterious magic that cannot be logically explained. *The assumption that a tumor disappears only by some fluke of magic is misguided.* The credit must be given to the body and its incredible power to heal itself.

Valerie found out that healing is hard but worthwhile work. Going through a natural healing process is rewarding, life-affirming and empowering. Self-healing improves self-image and motivation to live a fulfilling life, partially devoted to helping others.

Valerie is a vibrant, energetic woman who helps people lose weight with her own business. Her energy and excitement about her life is catchy. I was astounded by her ability to compile and implement the Alternative program that was so much like mine.

The Alternative approach to Cancer is rapidly gaining because it gets results.

The assumption that all we need to do is to throw more and more money at scientists looking through microscopes hoping to find a promising "cure" is one that has held us back and kept us in the dark for one-hundred years. The magic bullet may NEVER be found. Instead we need to learn how to heal our lives. We need to start early on with prevention. In this way we will conquer Cancer, not with a check but by keeping Cancer in check with a healthy lifestyle that supports rather than *taxes* our immune system!

"Human progress has never been achieved with unanimous consent. Those who are enlightened first are compelled to pursue the light in spite of others." This statement, made by Christopher Columbus in 1492 when he discovered the Americas and proved the world was not flat, has never been so true.

Another assumption we must question is that Mammograms are prevention. Mammography is a device for detection that actually causes the disease it seeks to identify. Radiation to a sensitive area of a woman's body may, over time, actually cause Breast Cancer. Thermography and blood tests, I believe, are the wave of the future. Self-exams are very important as a large percentage of women find the tumor themselves.

MEDICAL ADVANCES MUST BE QUESTIONED

The assumption that the Medical Establishment has made "progress" with "Medical advances" in Cancer has to be seriously questioned when we look at the last century. The mortality rate has not significantly decreased for most Cancers. Cancer kills one American every minute! One in two men and one in three women will get Cancer this year. Cancer, a rare disease in the early 1900s with doctors averaging two cases a year, is now a common occurrence.

It's time to change the basic paradigm the approach to Cancer has been based upon. The Cancer Industry is big business and has fed upon itself to monstrous proportions using outdated and antiquated treatments. Money has supplanted health in importance. We must reverse out priorities in order to make real progress. When eighty percent of people with Cancer who do the Medical treatment will die with or from the disease, we must look hard at what we are doing wrong. We must seriously question present methods of treating this disease and our whole approach in defining it. We must focus on the patient, instead of the tumor or other symptoms. We must admit that surgery, chemotherapy, and radiation do not always return the patient to good health.

The people in this text took control of their lives. They changed their diet, began a vigorous exercise routine, and looked hard at the stresses and distresses in their lives. They went into group therapy, began meditating, and doing visualization. They kept a journal or found other ways to express their feelings. They forgave others who had caused them pain. In addition they found ways to help others. They learned to laugh at their own foibles. They prayed and asked others to pray for them. They visualized and affirmed their goal of getting well.

THE CURE FOR Cancer IS WITHIN YOU

We must start looking at inner space. The "cure" is within all of us to turn Cancer back into glowing health. No drug or procedure can ever do a better job than our own immune and healing systems once they are supported. No cure "out there" can match the complex healing systems we have within. The intelligence of the body can heal us of most any disease including Cancer.

We would better spend our time, money and efforts learning how to care for our bodies, learning self-healing and what I call "self-lumpectomy." Mastectomies are being gradually phased out by lumpectomies. These soon, I hope, will be phased out by self-lumpectomies that require no surgery.

NEIL SEARCHES FOR A CURE

Neil Ruzic, a science writer and magazine publisher, was diagnosed with Mantle-cell Lymphoma in 1998. He refused chemotherapy which he refers to derisively as "Chemo-culture" and "Chemo-toxins" because of its acceptance as a "standard therapy" for most all Cancers despite its harmful, toxic effects on normal cells, damaging effects on the immune system, and only temporary results in eradicating Cancer cells.

Doing his own research, Neil found that Chemotherapy does not achieve positive results in Mantle-cell Lymphoma, although four doctors at leading Cancer Centers "demanded" that he submit to it. He also refused radiation. He did submit to surgery—a removal of his enlarged spleen. This is a crucial part of the lymphatic system as are the lymph nodes, lymphatic vessels, tonsils, adenoids, appendix, and perhaps even the liver. He was "given" two years to live.

He subsequently wrote the book, *Racing to a Cure: A Cancer Victim Refuses Chemotherapy and Finds Tomorrow's Cures in Today's Scientific Laboratories.*

In this book, Neil relates about being a science writer and having a plane as well as unlimited funds, traveling the world seeking "scientific cures" such as vaccines made out of the patient's own tumor cells. Most oncologists told him he could not try any new immune-supportive therapies unless he had "twice-failed chemotherapy."

In other words, as he points out, the failure of chemotherapy drugs is blamed on the patient! This from a Medical viewpoint that so resists a patient taking responsibility for his or her Cancer because it might induce some blame and guilt! He was urged to start Chemotherapy in three months or he would die. Four major Cancer Centers in the U.S. gave him this ultimatum.

Although Neil has a disdain of the "mystical world of Alternative Medicine," writing it off as useless, he actually incorporated many of its practices while flying around the country looking for a non-toxic, biological "Cure" which he was sure he would find if he went on an exhaustive search of top scientific labs, leaving no stone unturned! From his new vigorous goal of research and interviews to find his own solutions, though always exclusively through a scientific viewpoint, his symptoms abate, his lymph nodes stop growing and even begin shrinking! This happens five months after his splenectomy without any other therapy whatsoever. His own immune and healing systems, claiming no credit, went quietly about their job of self-healing while he was desperately searching "out there" for the magic Cure.

Neil continued to refuse the recommended Chemotherapy. He saw the damage it did to the patient, its temporary remission record, and its ineffectiveness for his type of Cancer. Meanwhile, his friend Ellen opted for a bone-marrow transplant at the City of Hope for her Mantle Cell Lymphoma, and the high-dose Chemotherapy opens her up to an infection that kills her.

One scientist told him point blank, "Here's my advice: don't attack your Lymphoma until it starts growing. Don't disrupt whatever equilibrium you have achieved—even with immunology, even with a vaccine. I have one patient with Mantle-Cell Lymphoma like yours who has been in remission for sixteen years!"

After seven months without any therapy whatsoever, his Lymphoma was still "indolent." After a year, only one lymph node had gotten larger. Opinions he got where not surprisingly that the vaccinators suggested making a vaccine, the radiation experts said to irradiate, and the surgeon suggested cutting.

Neil was determined, by hook or crook, to find that illusive Cure in the biotech labs around the country. Four years into his search, without any therapy or Chemo, his disease had stabilized. Could it be the Celebrex he decided to take? But no doctor would give the arthritis drug credit. The doctors were perplexed. Why was this patient doing so well without any Chemotherapy?

After four years, he did have a relapse. He had found a biological immune booster, Rituxan, which solves his problem.

He calls this a Cure. *Why he can't give his immune system credit is beyond my comprehension.*

Neil is a hard-driving achiever. He rejected "Alternative Medicine" because his brother died after almost starving himself to death on an ultra-minimal vegetarian diet. His brother was also a high achiever, putting pressure on himself to graduate from Medical School at age twenty.

Could the distress of his brother's death have been the emotional loss that contributed to Neil's Cancer? He doesn't connect stress to Cancer. Yet he does write about it.

"If my treatment was to be something other than Chemo, there wasn't time to find a Cure. I was desperate. In the past whenever I've been stressed, I have sought refuge in work, thereby subjugating worry to overcoming the problem that produced the anxiety in the first place. It has been that way in launching my magazines and in battling the Bahamian government to continue the science island. (He was so successful he bought an island and turned it into a science preserve!) Striving. Fighting. Turning liabilities into assets."

Learning to meditate might help him remain Cancer free. His high stress life, flying around the country, pressuring himself to find that elusive Cure, certainly doesn't create the most healing environment. On the other hand, he seemed to take tremendous pleasure in flying his plane, which he calls "Papa Whiskey." Neil even used the plane's engine sound to achieve a meditative state: "I lapsed into an electric quiet as if the vibrations from a long flight in Papa Whiskey were still murmuring in my bones."

Neil is a wonderful writer, yet reading this tale of frenetic search left me exhausted! Still, and without fanfare, his body steadfastly went on its own healing flight.

A hard look at what Neil actually did to help his body heal is most revealing:

1. He took control of his own healing program, refusing destructive Chemotherapy and radiation, only submitting to surgery to excise his enlarged spleen.

2. He began an exercise program including swimming fifty laps and alternating with ten-mile bike rides through the forest.

3. He changed his diet to "slow food", whatever that means! He carefully omitted diet and nutrition information calling green tea a "pipe dream." He did find out that grape skins contain resveratrol, which metabolizes into the anti-Leukemic agent picatannol, thus finding science in Nature.

4. He dedicated his life to helping others with Mantle-Cell Lymphoma, starting e-mail chains.

5. He used his creative writing ability to aid his healing.

6. He had a good marriage to buffer him emotionally and lend support at every stage.

7. Neil visualized himself well when he finally would be able to find the scientific "Cure."

8. He prayed and had others pray for him "just in case."

Still, Neil insisted on that "scientific cure" manufactured by a pharmaceutical company. His assumption that this would be the one and only way he could get well confused and misled him. The exciting research into the immune system that he found in this new world of self-discovery is not what interests him. **But the truth is his body healed itself.**

THE TALENTED WILL SURVIVE

The assumption that if we are talented we are above having to worry about our health has been disproved many times. Steven Sprouse died at age fifty of Lung Cancer and Heart Failure in a hospital in New York City. A brilliant dress designer, artist, and photographer, Stephen became the "darling of fashion" with spare, colorful dress designs in the early eighties. However, his business acumen never matched his creativity.

A photo of Stephen with the creative director of *Vanity Fair* at an art gallery opening shows a cherubic-faced, intense, longhaired man with a funny hat over a headband and a designer jacket. He has a big, dimpled smile on his face with intense, dark eyes.

What happened to this creative, vital man who literally pops off the newsprint page with his vital energy and enthusiasm for life? The obituary explains that his first two collections were huge successes. However, he was out of business from 1985 to 1987. What despair and hopelessness did he feel from this roller-coaster financial ride?

In 1987, he again opened shops in New York and at the Beverly Center in Los Angeles, but lacked financial backing and closed down again, this time for four years from 1988 to

1992. Yet his line was good enough to be carried by Bergdorf-Goodman and Barneys, New York in 1995.

Despite such commercial ups and downs (standard issue for most creative artists), Stephen's talent was so admired that his designs continued to fetch high prices in vintage stores after his production halted.

A movie, based on the book, *Slaves of New York,* by Tama Janowitz shows the character "Wilfredo" chain-smoking, wearing his train conductor hat and black-on-black outfit. This character was blatantly patterned after Sprouse.

A businessman in New York explains his "failure" in the commercial fashion world. "If you make a couple of hot things and milk them, that's how you make money in this world. I don't think Stephen was really focused on being huge, making a lot of money. He was an idealist with an ideal collection. He never sold out."

Stephen followed his own muse, like most creative artists. Yet he was aware of what he must do to create success. "If Andy Warhol were alive today, he'd totally be doing stuff for Target," he admitted. Yet this type of success was what he rejected. He always used very expensive fabric and the clothing was so beautifully made that anyone could wear it in style. It always looked elegant.

What lifestyle factors contributed to his way too early death? Certainly, the chain smoking. But how about the financial distress, the roller-coaster that this sensitive, creative genius endured in being true to his vision while ignoring his business survival? My guess is that this combination of cigarettes and financial ruin following on the heals of huge successes and the feelings of despair this must have engendered, led to his Lung Cancer at age forty-nine. The hospital he went to may have given him Chemotherapy, which may have contributed to his death of heart failure as Chemotherapy has been proven to damage the heart.

Of course, this is only my guess. But perhaps Stephen would be alive today if he had quit smoking, gone on a detox and de-stress program, while learning to better manage his finances. (*Los Angeles. Times* Obituaries, March 6, 2004).

ATTACKING CANCER WITH DESTRUCTIVE TREATMENTS IS WRONG

We can heal naturally from many diseases. I believe Cancer is one of them. When we give up the assumption that attacking Cancer cells and tumors with a war-like approach will eradicate them and we will then automatically regain our health, we will find a better approach.

Cancer is a degeneration of the mind, body, and spirit. When we give up focusing on tumors and Cancer cells and instead see the whole picture—the patient is a sick, dispirited and perhaps a very depressed person, possibly overloaded with toxins, who needs to get well, we will indeed see "advances" in medicine.

This shift in paradigm, this new perspective will yield the results we are searching for. *We must give up the assumption that if only we can find a "Cure" out there, that "Cure" will solve all our problems.*

Creating health is the best road back to wellness for anyone with Cancer. When you take the first step, the determination to get well and take responsibility to accomplish it, the body will hear the message and immediately begin to respond. You only need to make that decision and then follow through. Health is on the way!

CHAPTER 27

The Good News—You Can Get Well from Cancer Using Entirely Natural Means

THERE IS A way to get well from Cancer. It does not entail destroying Cancer cells and tumors with mutilating surgery, cytotoxic drugs and carcinogenic radiation. It does not even depend on the surgical removal of tumors. The way to get well from Cancer is to make a concerted, focused daily effort to bring your health back up to normal: physically, mentally, spiritually, and most of all emotionally. The body will not need tumors when you regain your health and your will to live. The body with your will power and healing lifestyle program will either discard tumors or steadily shrink them. They may also just stop growing, becoming non-threatening to the body or "indolent."

Taking responsibility for your own healing is the first step in turning on your immune system and telling it to get back to work! The brain is the Master-commander of the immune system. If you have been thinking that there is no more reason to live, that your life feels hopeless, that you cannot get through the traumas and down-turns in your life, that you "wish you were dead," that your life is "stuck," a tumor is a reminder to find reasons to live. **Cancer is a communication directly to you—you have to change your life.**

Your body can no longer take the kinds of pressures you are putting on it and cannot deal with the toxins you are exposing it to mentally, physically and emotionally without breaking down into serious, chronic disease.

GETTING WELL

Cancer gives you the opportunity to get into shape physically. It is also a reminder that toxic emotions such as suppressed anger and resentment, jealousy, guilt, fear and other negative emotions can make you very ill. Cancer is truly a gift to get your life back up to glowing health with daily caring for your body, mind, soul, and spirit. It is a tremendous reminder that we are here on earth to help others.

Others have found out how to get well naturally. You can do it too.

Kari, once a Breast Cancer patient, opted out of the Medical Treatment, the surgery, drugs, and radiation that were recommended, not only began to get well on the MOTEP program and taking the supplements that Dr. James Privitera recommended, even trained for the marathon. She reported glowing health and a full return of her energy, one year later after being diagnosed with a biopsy. She volunteered to help me out at speaking tours and was on my video at the Cancer Convention.

Five years later, she was still healthy! However, the tumor, though shrunken, was still in her breast. She decided on a drastic measure to get rid of the tumor. She tried bloodroot, called Black Salve. To me this was wrong. The tumor was still there for a reason. Her body was not yet ready to discard it. And as it wasn't interfering with her health or activities, I questioned this decision.

Kari used the salve. This was caustic and made a hole in her breast. "The hole won't close!" she reported. I shuddered to hear this negative result.

Her health began, once more, to go downhill. She then went into the hospital. The doctors could find no Breast Cancer cells in her breast! However, they found some in her bones. They began to radiate her.

"They gave her too much radiation!" her boyfriend Rob told me. It affected her lungs. She couldn't breathe. They then put her on oxygen. It was in the hospital setting that she lost her health. She died in 2007.

"Because of your program, she had five more precious years of wonderful living," Rob related to me over the phone. "If she had done the Medical treatment immediately she would have missed out on all those years. She finished the Marathon in five hours and fifty-five minutes. She was triumphant. I had never seen her so energetic and healthy."

Rob and I both celebrated the fact that Kari had extended and improved her life. Her impatience with her tumor was the beginning of the end. Dr. Privitera tells of patients who have lived twenty years with a tumor. We found out the hard way that the tumor is not the disease, only a symptom that the body needs to heal. This may take as much time as the body needs. The wisdom of the body cannot be questioned.

Orlan Wachter appeared on my video nine years after she was told she had three months to live when she was diagnosed with Breast, Colon, and Lung Cancer in exploratory surgery. She did not submit to the further surgery recommended to remove her breast, one of her lungs, and part of her colon with a colostomy bag. Instead Orlan went on the MOTEP program and also read every book she could lay her hands on that described what she could do for herself. She tried a lot of things and kept up what worked for her. In her seventies, she was busy with a schedule of work and travel.

I called her at work. Her enthusiasm for natural healing knows no bounds.

"You have to stop doing what is killing you," she advises. "You have to go on a gung-ho health program and retrieve your vital energies."

I call Orlan Wachter my star student. She had the worst-case scenario of anyone I've ever encountered. The doctor told her that Lung Cancer was "very aggressive" in women, thus the brief three-month prognosis even with the extensive surgery they recommended but she refused. She overcame the odds against her by taking the bull by the horns; taking responsibility and changing her life into comprehensive self-support and helping others get through Cancer. She has constantly volunteered to help other Cancer patients, appear on my videos, or speak at conferences.

Leila moved back to Northern California to take care of her mother. She is doing very well devoted to her new career in Alternative Medicine and has had no recurrence of her Cervical Cancer. She has a newfound sense of self and high self-esteem and virtually glows with good health and beauty.

Deirdre Morgan moved to Santa Fe, New Mexico where she has a busy career as a life-coach. On a recent visit to Pasadena, she did her group lecture in which she described a trip to Brazil where she worked with a Healer to resolve some old issues and unresolved emotions and pains from an automobile accident. She went through a healing crisis in which warts appeared on her arms and back where the excruciating pains had been. These warts were temporary and soon disappeared along with all of her pain. "Ageless" is a good description of the beautiful, energetic Deirdre, with her warmth and intelligence shining like the sun in the dark of the evening.

THE FUTURE OF CANCER TREATMENT

Political forces such as the FDA and The American Cancer Society can keep the pressure on to "treat" Cancer with toxic drugs, radiation, and surgery. However the future looks far different. The government is only as strong as "all the people."

When people, such as the examples in this book, do the research themselves and find out that the way to heal Cancer is to bolster the immune system rather than destroy it, they lead the way to the future of Cancer treatment. We will recognize Cancer for what it is, the depletion of the immune system because of toxic overload, distress and depression, and lack of self-care. We will prescribe, not drugs, but a program like MOTEP to heal the disease in a slow, methodical way. Hippocrates hospital was more like a spa. There were hot healing waters in a spiritual atmosphere with interpretation of dreams. A special healing diet was given. Hippocrates, the Father of Modern Medicine, actually prohibited surgery for Cancer because it was too traumatic for the body and didn't solve the problem.

THE FUTURE IS HERE

Four out of ten Americans spend some $23 billion annually on Alternative Cancer treatments. People recognize that conventional medical treatments are outmoded, archaic, carcinogenic, and life-threatening as well as prohibitively, astronomically expensive. They are looking for ways to help themselves.

A new study links breast radiotherapy to heart death risk. In Hamburg, Germany, researchers found an increased risk of dying from cardiovascular disease in 7,427 Breast Cancer patients, seventeen to seventy-one years old studied for fourteen years or more. Considerable damage to the heart was found especially when the left breast was treated with radiation. Overall a 2.2 fold increase was found in irradiated patients. (Reuters Internet News, March 18, 2004).

Yet radiation is prescribed for more and more Breast Cancer patients. (*New York Times*, "Debate on Radiation in Breast Cancer" 02/25/04).

Cancer patients are not given full information on options by their doctors and oncologists. It was found in the Netherlands that doctors discuss palliative Chemotherapy designed to shrink tumors even when a cure is unlikely. Less than half of the patients are told about "watchful-waiting" which involves treating symptoms as they develop rather than using Chemo to attack a tumor. **In metastasized Cancer, watchful waiting and palliative chemotherapy were found to have similar survival rates. The oncologists discussed quality of life in less than half of the patients!**

Even Neil Ruzic, who disdained Alternative medicine labeling it "alternatoid" medicine, admitted that herbs sometimes help: "Most herbs are safe, and some such as saw palmetto, which relieves the advance of benign enlarged prostates, and antioxidants which can help prevent macular and other degeneration are entering mainstream medicine. If you determine that an herbal medicine will do no harm and that it has some basis in science, why not try it for prevention?"

MIND-BODY MEDICINE COMES OF AGE

We live in an enlightened time. Mind-body medicine or psychoneuroimmunology, is a recognized and accepted modality. Our thoughts and feelings contribute greatly to our health and well-being. Even boredom is bad for your health! It is now accepted that every disease has a psychosomatic component. Finding your distresses and stresses and working to ease them by creating new healing situations for yourself and others, will bolster your immune system and get it working in high gear again. The immune and healing systems are sophisticated, wise, and are the key to getting well from Cancer.

Neil found that there were four thousand genes in his Mantle Cell Lymphoma that had expression, and three thousand that did not. He picked one at random and asked what it showed.

"Well it means your interleukin-1 level is high, as you would expect in Lymphoma. IL-1 originates in macrophages during the early, nonspecific phase of an immune response. It's one of the fever-inducing molecules," a scientist in Los Angeles, Phil Koeffler told him.

I found that my body induced a specific loco-regional fever in my affected left breast when it turned red, hot, and stone-like during my self-healing process. Fever is one of the basic tools the body uses to heal disease. Think of sterilizing a bottle of fruit when canning it by dropping the sealed bottle in a hot bath of boiling water. This sterilizes out the germs and bacteria. The body utilizes this same basic tool—intense heat to sterilize out the germs, viruses, bacteria, and Cancer cells. It utilizes inflammation to cordon off the area to be repaired and healed. **We must not fear fever and inflammation and give drugs to combat them**. The body needs to use these tools to do its repair and healing work.

This healing reaction takes place when the body is sufficiently de-toxified and de-stressed. When a feeling of peace and calm is generated throughout the mind and body, and toxins are eliminated through a high-fiber, low-fat diet, the body can then get into its self-healing work. *Your body knows how to heal Cancer.* You need only to support it in every possible way.

The future of Cancer treatment lies in supporting rather than destroying the body's healing systems so the patient can get well and stay well.

CHAPTER 28

A Time-Capsule Journey to Cancer Centers of America 2525 A.D.

(The following is a fictional account)

RON JONES, THE founder of his own company, SongPro, developed Gastric Cancer four years after a lawsuit was filed against him. He had the idea of turning an electronic game-player into an audio and video receiver and applied to be a licensee to Game-Player International. They denied his application and sued him for infringement of intellectual property rights as he already had developed a web site for his new product.

A wonderfully inventive and creative black man, Ron had worked his way out of the ghetto of South-Central Los Angeles with his computer devices, printer improvements, and other high-tech innovations and inventions. He was always coming up with ways to enhance and expand existing technologies using a creative intelligence that never missed a beat. A sunny, happy person, he was voted "Entrepreneur of the Year" by the New York Interracial Council for Business.

Game-Player International eventually reached a settlement with Ron and awarded him a license, but by then he was already ill. "You can educate yourself and try to beat or work within the system," he said, "but the corporate world is powerful and try to block your progress at every turn."

Also in Los Angeles, Sharon Dubois, a beautiful blonde forty-eight year old woman, obviously in the prime of her life, was left by her husband of almost twenty years. Alfred had an affair with his young secretary that developed into a serious relationship. He eventually divorced Sharon, who was shocked and pleaded with him to try to save their marriage. Sharon still loved him with all her heart. She had worked diligently on her appearance even going for plastic surgery, to try to keep her handsome husband coming home to her. Her belief was that if she was able to stave off the aging process enough, she could avoid such a betrayal and loss.

Sharon also bought a new wardrobe of designer clothing and silky lingerie. But nothing worked. When Alfred left for good, she was inconsolable and cried her eyes out for weeks and months at a time. Two years later, still grieving, Sharon found a lump in her breast while bathing in the shower. Upon a biopsy, a Cancer diagnosis was given to her by a Surgical Oncologist.

Ron and Sharon met at the hospital where doctors offered them both a New Clinical Trial of the Future. They were offered a trip in a specially equipped time-travel rocket ship to sample what Cancer Treatment Center of America could offer them in the year 2525, five hundred plus years from now.

Both agreed to this breathtakingly exciting trial.

"I'm so glad to meet you," Ron greeted Sharon who brightened upon seeing this congenial black man with his impish grin. They were to meet on Tuesday wearing special space suits they were given at the Biomedical Laboratories in Culver City, Astroglide Inc., located on Washington Boulevard.

"This is a very special opportunity to learn about what the future holds for all people world-wide who develop Cancer!" Sharon pointed out. Ron agreed enthusiastically, always the inventor and tremendously curious about new advances in Medical Treatment and Science.

RON AND SHARON TAKE OFF

On Tuesday, with much anticipation, they drove to the Time-Capsule site in Culver City where a big, vacant lot next to Astroglide Inc. held the sleek rocket ship. They were a little nervous. They would be the first patients ever with Cancer to time-travel for a clinical trial. There were photographers on hand to record the event. It subsequently made the front page of all the newspapers.

Peeking inside the rocket ship, Sharon saw an interior completely covered in soft, padded gray felt. She guessed that this would help absorb any shock they would encounter as they leaped ahead over five hundred years. Gingerly, she took a seat on a cushioned, gray felt covered bench. Ron soon joined her, sitting besides Sharon.

He could see she was anxious and nervous, so Ron gently took her hand. Sharon gratefully let her hand linger in his as the engines started up full-throttle! There was a great roar and then a loud whine. Sharon closed her eyes and even said a little prayer, though she was not usually a religious person. What would the future look like? Would the doctors of the future still recommend a mastectomy? She felt strongly that she needed her breasts to attract a new lover, and perhaps even a second husband.

Ron was queasy, but excited. The prognosis of his Stomach Cancer had been "terminal in three months." Ron was still in his forties and felt he had a full, inventive life ahead of him. He already had ideas for cell-phones, perhaps converting them into video cameras. At the least he wanted cell phones to be visual TV phones so you could view the person you were talking to. He had an idea about how to go about implementing this new technology. He was already starting to program the scheme in his head.

CANCER CENTER OF THE FUTURE

After an interminable twenty-four hours, the felt parted and the large door slid open with a whizzing noise. In front of them was a huge temple-like white building with the sign, "Cancer Treatment Centers of America" emblazoned on the front. As Ron and Sharon stepped out of the Time-Travel Rocket Ship, they were greeted by Althea, a warm and gracious Nurse Practitioner.

"Welcome to the future of Cancer Treatment," she said smiling. "We are very happy you were brave enough to refuse outmoded and archaic 2008 Cancer treatments and time travel to see us. Many things have changed in regard to this most feared disease that used to be considered 'terminal'. Of course, we still don't have one hundred percent of our patients get well, but most of them do. We have about a ninety-five percent healing-rate for all types of Cancer, and most people who come here not only get well but often start new careers helping others to understand, prevent and heal Cancer."

"Have you found the Cure for Cancer?" Ron asked anxiously. "We've spent billions of dollars looking for it since the year 1971 when Richard Nixon declared the War on Cancer. Did you find it at last in the Scientific Biomedical Laboratories?"

Althea smiled knowingly, "Yes, you wasted a lot of time and money looking for a magical substance, a wonder drug, some chemical that would erase years of damage to your body. What we found, in fact, is that there is no 'Cure.' "

Sharon looked confused. "Then why have I come all this way, risking my life to time-travel all the way to you?"

Althea laughed. "We will help you to learn how to heal your Breast Cancer. By the way, we will also help you to prevent recurrence. You will then be able to teach others that are stuck back in the 'Standard, Conventional' treatment back in 2008. Those so-called treatments were outmoded back in 1940, but the political and economic forces stymied any changes. However, there was a consumer revolt in the nineties or even sooner. People began demanding what was then called 'Alternative Medicine.' But it really was natural healing, the only way to absolutely get well from Cancer."

"You mean we won't be given any toxic chemicals, burning radiation, or mutilating surgeries?" Ron asked.

"Of course not!"

"Well, then, how will we overcome Cancer?" Ron was aghast and confused. He wanted a quick fix, the magic bullet he was sure he would find in this hospital of the future.

"Let me show you around our Center," Althea continued, unphased.

They walked through a huge doorway. What they saw took their breath away.

The Center overlooked a very large, intense turquoise lake that could be seen through wall-sized picture windows. Sharon's anxiety seemed to be slipping away as she gazed upon the magnificent blue body of water. It certainly was a healing atmosphere here. Not like the cold, sterile hospital Sharon thought she would end up in.

From the Welcoming Hall, they moved through corridors with large abstract paintings on the walls, full of color and light, to the gym. There were weights, exercise machines, and slant-boards for sit-ups. There were treadmills and a team of personal trainers. Cancer patients were striving to work out as hard as they possibly could. Even the pale ones, who could only slowly do a sit-up, smiled back.

Through the exercise room, they entered a locker-room and then onto an Olympic-size pool. There were swimmers, water walkers, and water aerobicizers. Everyone seemed to be having a great time.

"But all this is," Ron commented, "is a gym!" He couldn't fathom the reason for this in a Cancer hospital. He had pictured lines of beds for patients, with lots of tubes for infusions of some sort of drug. "What is this for?" Ron demanded.

Althea smiled again. "Did you know that when you exercise you sweat out toxins that could have contributed to your Cancer. Also did you know that oxygen kills Cancer cells? It's better than any drug. Cancer cells cannot survive in an oxygenated internal environment. Otto Warburg discovered that fact at least a century ago. They gave him the Nobel prize."

Sharon looked awed. "I didn't know you could destroy Cancer cells simply by exercising!"

Althea nodded and then led them to a sauna. "Heat also destroys Cancer cells. Here you can sweat out toxins, relax, and help the body create its own fever-healing reaction. Instead of bringing fever down, as we used to do in fear, we encourage the body to create heat. Instead of anti-inflammatory drugs, we try to induce an inflammatory reaction in which the body uses white blood cells to wall off the tumor so the heat and cytokines, 'cells that move,' can bombard and destroy it."

Sharon still looked dubious. This certainly seemed "ordinary" treatment compared to drastic, dramatic, and gruesome mastectomies. The drama was all internal. Certainly, she wanted to keep her breasts! But this seemed anything but "futuristic." She had expected technology, CAT-scans, a science lab complete with white-coated scientists looking under microscopes, Frankenstein's laboratory, Bio-Tech Gene Wonder Drugs, glistening test tubes and huge, sparkling machinery. Even Cancer-curing robots performing "robotic surgery."

"Let's continue the tour," Althea said softly, breaking Sharon's trance.

They came to a room where the occupants were sitting on the floor, their legs folded and their arms resting upon them. They were quiet. You could almost hear them breathe. Althea put her finger to her lips and they walked on. They came to a chapel where everyone was praying. Ron and Sharon knelt and pressed their hands together, so anxious were they to join this group of worshippers. "Oh, God, please help me to get well," Sharon prayed. "Please let me know I am in the right place to accomplish this huge task!" Tears came into her eyes. But then, surprisingly, stunningly Sharon knew she was in the right place. A feeling of wonder came over her. Ron felt awe and wonder too, as if granted a great gift and opportunity.

After a while, Althea tapped their shoulders and they moved on. In another room, people chanted to a Gohonzon. "These people practice Buddhism," she pointed out. Chanting is a form of verbal prayer with a mantra, in this case they say, "Nam Myoho Renge Kyo" and recite the Lotus Sutra. Most of them visualize their healing while they chant. They "see" themselves healthy and well. They visualize little lions eating their Cancer cells, or Pac-men gobbling them up. The aggressive types visualize "smart-bombs" destroying their Cancer cells. Everyone is encouraged to dream up his or her own scenario. The creative process is very helpful in Cancer healing. We want you to learn to create your own health."

Ron, a super-creative person, nodded. He understood the value of creating, but creating health with his imagination and artistic abilities was something new to him. Yet it was beginning to make sense. It had the ring of truth. He smiled knowingly.

The next large room was a cafeteria. Both Sharon and Ron said, "I'm hungry!" simultaneously. It had been a long trip through all those years!"

They noticed juice bars. There was a menu of juices: carrot, carrot-apple, carrot-orange, carrot-garlic, and carrot-celery. There were beet and beet with greens mixtures. Other green juices such as cucumber-watercress, spinach and cabbage with garlic, wheat-grass with apple to make it more palatable, and many other green combinations, some mixed with radish, ginger, garlic, and fresh dill, were displayed.

Both Ron and Sharon ordered glasses of fresh vegetable juices and drank them up without further hesitation. They went down smoothly. "I feel better already!" Ron joked. He still wondered what he was doing here and where was the "Cure"?

"We can stop for lunch," Althea beckoned them. Sharon noticed a line-up of woks, steamers, and a display of fresh salads with many types of greens: watercress, spinach, romaine lettuce, cucumber, green and red onions, and herbs such as oregano, thyme, basil, dill and rosemary. Dressings were listed as flaxseed oil or Extra-virgin olive oil with garlic, lemon, balsamic vinegar, rice vinegar, or apple-cider vinegar.

Sharon and Ron ordered salads. They then went on to the main course buffet. Here was featured piles of barley, brown rice, and other whole grains and beans combined with a medley of vegetables such as zucchini, carrots, red bell-pepper, green beans, peas, cabbage, brussel sprouts, broccoli, and tomatoes. They heaped these stews on their plates. They also opted for fresh steamed salmon enhanced with garlic, lemon, and rosemary.

For dessert there were fresh fruit cups, mixed seasonal fruits including cantaloupe balls, mango chunks, apples, pears and berries. This was served with Cinnamon Graham crackers made with honey and a pot of hot, green tea.

"This is great food," Ron complimented Althea, but can it help cure Cancer?"

Althea nodded. "These foods are rich in Beta-carotene, Laetrile or Vitamin B-17, Omega Three fatty acids, and fiber. All these nutrients have proven scientific records of preventing and reversing Cancer."

Her all-knowingness perplexed Ron, and Sharon started to question it.

"O.K.," she said. I admit that my diet wasn't so hot. After Alfred left, I didn't care what I ate. In fact I often stuffed myself, splurging on cakes, cookies, pastries, steaks, hamburgers, and French fries, washed down with cokes, anything to feel better. I even started to gain weight!"

I was too busy to eat right," Ron admitted. "I would just go to a fast-food joint or greasy spoon and swallow some high-fat junk like three-cheese pizza with a diet cola so I wouldn't gain weight."

"You both were overloaded with saturated fats, preservatives, and other toxins. This may very well have contributed to your breakdown into Cancer," Althea noted. "Also you ate too much meat and sugar, and probably worthless white flour too."

"Yes, I started my day often with doughnuts," Sharon admitted. "I washed them down with lots of cups of coffee."

Althea shook her head. "You are lucky you are still here. Let's finish eating our nourishing, detoxifying lunch and then continue our tour. We also provide Vitamin and mineral supplementation. We serve Essiac tea, formulated from an old Indian recipe for aiding people with Cancer. It was discovered and developed by Rene Caisse, a Canadian. Essiac is her name spelled backwards.

Ron and Sharon smiled. This was starting to make sense.

SUPPORTING YOUR IMMUNE SYSTEM
IS THE KEY TO CONQUERING CANCER

After lunch they headed for a tour of the outdoor spa. It was a wonderful, sunny day and Lake Lotus glistened in the sun. "We do morning hikes around the lake and deep-breathing exercises like Tai Chi and Yoga, bringing our mats down near the water. We also encourage lake swimming for the bolder patients, although most, I admit, opt for the Olympic-size heated indoor pool. But here near the center, you will also note these smaller pools of hot water," she gestured as they walked past. There was a line-up of natural mineral water hot-pools, sulphur baths, and clay pools for mineral rich "mud."

"Fortunately, our spa is located over natural mineral hot-water veins from deep within the earth. This water has been used for centuries in healing disease, pain, fatigue, and for general rejuvenation and detoxification."

Ron noted that some of these pools were hot enough to generate a steamy atmosphere above them. He breathed in the steam and found it deeply refreshing.

Althea went on with her informative tour. "Both oxygen and heat kill Cancer cells more efficiently than toxic Chemotherapy drugs, hormone treatments, radiation, and even surgery that you used as 'standard' treatment back in 2008. Oxygen and heat also do not have adverse side effects when used correctly. We don't advocate sitting in hot tubs or the saunas for more than ten or fifteen minutes at a time.

"Remember, overdoing or 'high-dose' anything is dangerous. That is why they eliminated, finally, Autologous bone-marrow transplants for Breast Cancer. This procedure used high-dose Chemotherapy, which proved way too toxic for a patient who already had their stem cells removed and frozen. These were to be injected later to 'rescue' the patient. Unfortunately, the toxicity and immune destroying high-dose drugs proved to be overkill. The patient often died of infections, as their immune system was totally wiped out. Also the Cancer, without the immune system fiercely guarding it, often metastasized wildly out of control afterward."

Ron and Sharon were beginning to comprehend this strange new treatment for Cancer in the year 2525. "I think I am beginning to understand," Sharon gestured with her hands. "We used to aim for aggressively attacking and killing the Cancer. We felt it needed to be surgically removed and that doctors could 'get it all.' But you are working, instead, on rebuilding our health that has deteriorated from lack of care, exposure to toxins, and traumatic emotional and financial loss, all causing extreme stress and general deterioration!"

"That's exactly right. You hit the nail right on the head," Althea said. "Congratulations, I think you understand our 'futuristic' approach to Cancer. When you really think about it, killing the Cancer cells with toxic drugs, dangerous surgeries, and carcinogenic radiation doesn't resonate because it doesn't take into account the fact that the person is extremely ill. These treatments you had back then mostly added to further destruction, deterioration, and more disease. We consider Cancer patients to be in a state of steeply declining health, often with a weakened will to live, and we work on all levels—spiritual, physical, mental, and emotional to bring that person's well being back to them. We build up the immune system, instead of tearing it down. To put it simply, we are here to help you re-build your health from square one!"

"That makes sense," Ron nodded. "It's all so clear, I wonder why we didn't see it back then."

"I think that you panicked when a diagnosis of Cancer was made. Oncologists thought "aggressive" treatment to kill Cancer cells would work. They saw the Cancer cells as 'termites' invading the body that needed to be exhumed and destroyed. Today we see Cancer cells as weak, damaged cells. The immune system is quite capable of cleaning them out, or even restoring them to health without toxic and destructive treatments. We encourage wellness here. A healthy body will not permit Cancer cells to grow. Experiments to inject Cancer cells into healthy people are a total failure. We also work on the all-important Will to Live."

WHAT DOES IT TAKE TO GET WELL?

They entered the Center again after visiting the hot pools with views of the lake. "This room is for group therapy," Althea motioned.

Sharon opened the front door and heard a woman crying. "And then my husband disappeared," she sobbed. "I found out later that he ran off with a young actress in his new movie."

Sharon sat down next to the woman and cradled her. "Almost the exact same thing happened to me, only it was the proverbial, young secretary," she said, comforting the woman by rocking her.

The woman looked startled at first. Then the two nodded and cried together. "Two years later I had Breast Cancer," Sharon related. "I was diagnosed with Endometrial Cancer two years later," the woman whose name was Faith, agreed.

"We can help each other get well," Sharon volunteered.

Faith nodded, anxious for a partner in her misery.

Ron sat down. When it was his turn in the circle of partic-ipants, he told them about his hard struggle to be innovative in a rigid, structured corporate environment. "You see I had so many new ideas. But these corporate cats, well, they don't want any infringement on their intellectual properties. They finally accepted the idea I had, but first they had to initiate a lawsuit. I was really blue, so depressed I had a hard time getting up in the morning. I knew that my idea was great and that they were wrong to turn me into an intellectual thief when I was only trying to help them by expanding and improving their products."

"How long after that were you diagnosed with Cancer?" Wally asked. "I was diagnosed with Colorectal Cancer after my business partner ran off with all the funds in our bank account. It took about two years of shock and sadness before I wound up sick." Wally hunched over in agony.

"Yes," Ron agreed. "That was about the same time for me. I was so tired of fighting 'the powers that be'. And I'm not one to be easily discouraged, either. But being labeled a com-mon thief was too much for me, I guess. I was just trying to explore my creative ability and improve my business and for that I was duly and severely punished."

Althea left for an hour while Sharon and Ron talked about their frustrations and disappointments with the oth-ers in the group. There wasn't a single one in the circle who had not had a major setback or death of a loved one before they developed some type of Cancer. There also was not one dry-eye in the group.

SLEEP CONTRIBUTES TO WELLNESS

After the hour was up, Althea returned. They then walked down the halls to the private rooms. "I'll show you your suites," Althea smiled. They were led to rooms designed like the time capsule with soft gray felt interiors, and beds covered in warm gray flannel blankets and gray goose-down comforters. There was no TV, only a stereo that played soft, soothing music. Colorful art adorned the walls. There was a closet for their clothes, a bathroom with a large bathtub and shower, and a bookcase full of books on healing, such as how to do guided imagery and visualization, Chinese herbs, Vitamin Therapy, and general books on healing Cancer naturally. One of the authors, Sharon noted, was Norman Cousins who advised people to laugh themselves well.

Each apartment had a terrace with tables and chairs overlooking the lake outside the kitchen.

"We encourage you to put in serious sleep-time. Eight-to-ten hours while you are getting well is minimum. You can also come here after lunch and take a siesta, or retire here anytime you feel tired or want to be alone. We have Science behind the benefits of sleep. Dr. David Spiegel at Stanford pointed out that sleep affects hormone levels—the important two: Melatonin and Cortisol. Melatonin pumped out during sleep acts as an antioxidant and slows estrogen production. Cortisol reaches its highest level in the dawn and declines during the day. That is except when we are under heavy stress, even if it is imagined. Then we have a rush of that stress hormone.

"Cortisol helps regulate immune activity, especially NK or Natural Killer Cells you need to destroy Cancer cells.

However, when you are under stress, the immune system is actually inactivated while your body works with adrenaline production in a 'fight-or-flight' state. Your body has only so much energy, and under stress it has to redirect its activities toward resolving threats, real situations or ones that are only imagined and worried about. Estrogen is also pumped out during stress."

"That makes sense," Sharon agreed. "My Breast Cancer is estrogen-dependent."

"Sleep will help regulate that excess estrogen back to a normal level," Althea told her. "Whole grains like barley and brown rice that we serve for lunch and at dinner will help you to eliminate excess estrogen also."

"All this makes so much common sense. But how will it work to obliterate my Cancer?" Ron asked.

"After you have spent around a month here, your body may go into a healing reaction or Crisis. You may experience fever, cells buzzing around like bees, inflammation and itching. Maybe even temporary paralysis of limbs or body parts."

Ron looked scared.

"Don't be frightened. The body needs a Crisis, usually, to heal. It's part of the healing system's job. It usually is a very temporary situation, in some cases only lasting a day or two. Everyone is different. For some, the tumor may just continue to get smaller and shrink in size until it finally disappears, or white cell count will decline in cases of leukemia and lymphoma when we have an overabundance of them."

"How do we cope with that trauma?" Sharon asked.

"We are here to support you. You will exercise through it, like relaxing swimming, and sitting in the hot tubs and sauna to actually encourage the fever-reaction. You will have massages. The fever is how the body 'burns out' the Cancerous cells."

"After that reaction, we will be well?" Ron asked.

"Not completely. You took two years to get sick you estimated, remember? It will take time to get well. You have to do the work to rebuild your body back to health. That is what the weights and exercise machines help you to do. The nourishing, special diet, vitamins, group therapy, yoga, hiking, and deep breathing all contribute. We have massage rooms here also with healing oils and herbs. This all works together to restore your health and vitality.

HAVING FUN CONTRIBUTES TO WELLNESS

"Let me show you the auditorium and screening room," Althea continued. They were led to a large theater with deep maroon velvet drapes covering a wide screen.

"We also have fun evenings of comedy, movies, amateur comedy nights where you get up to the mike and laugh at yourself and your foibles, and smile a lot. This sends endorphins to your brain, which carry a healing message. These are playful, entertaining evenings when you can forget that you are ill and just enjoy yourself. Believe it or not, having fun is part of the treatment! Even the Medical literature in your day and age states that, 'Generally happy people do not get Cancer.'

"But to answer your question, after the healing crisis, your body will usually discard and destroy tumors within a few weeks. Sometimes the tumor does stay in the body, however, even while you get well. We found that you can live for decades with some sign of the tumor still in your body while you feel well. That's the irony. You used to think getting the tumor out was the solution. However, removing the tumor does not make you well.

We ask you to stay here for four months. It's up to you, but a full nine months is optimum."

"Then we go back to Earth?" Ron inquired.

Althea laughed. "You are on Earth! Only you leaped ahead over five hundred years. Yes, you will go back to 2008. But you, hopefully, will take your new habits with you, the diet, the exercise, the sleep habits, and the ability to talk about your distresses and frustrations with others. You will see that it's important to express your anger in healthy ways, stand up for yourself, and count your blessings. You will better be able to review your life and make healthy decisions. Self-destructive habits will probably look a lot less appealing. Destructive relationships full of conflict and pain will either turn around, become positive and nurturing, or end. Most of all, you will have plenty of knowledge about Cancer healing so that you can help others get well too."

"I am so ready to try this approach!" Sharon enthused. "It seems like the only way to really get well from Cancer. But what about recurrence? That really frightens me."

"As long as you keep up this program, recurrence is not likely. You remember that the immune system has a memory. For instance, if you have Chicken Pox as a child, you usually will not go through it again as an adult. The immune system, after a total natural healing, will be stronger and savvier, if you will, once you have healed. Remember: Cancer is a state of toxicity and depression that overloads and inactivates the immune system.

"Say you encounter another big stress. Someone you love

deeply dies, for instance. Now you have new tools to defend yourself from more Cancer or heart problems. You organize a group therapy session with friends, maybe bringing a potluck dinner, so you can express your feelings. You join a YMCA and do weights, swimming, yoga, or whatever exercise you enjoy. You use a sauna there. Perhaps you visit a mineral-water spa. You make relaxing vacations an integral part of your routine. You keep up the mostly whole-grain, fruit and vegetable with juicing diet and take supplements. You put in extra sleep time.

"Maybe you take up writing a journal, write a book, do a painting, join a chorus, learn a musical instrument, start ballroom or square dancing, start any creative activity that you can get involved in from cooking to decorating. Adopt a cat or dog from the pound; animals can help you get out of yourself and your problems, substituting love and joy. You can chant, meditate, pray, and visualize whenever you find yourself falling into a negative mind-set. You work on positive relationships in your life and help those who have trouble forming them. You make a new friend. Everything you learn here at the Cancer Center will help you maintain your health when you return back to your own year."

"Then prevention is more about a lifestyle and how you feel about your life," Sharon noted. "I guess it means you find absorbing activities other than feeling sorry for yourself."

Althea nodded. "Yes, the mind-body connection is of the utmost importance in this disease. I would even say the Spirit is first!"

Ron nodded enthusiastically. "I dig this place already," he said grinning. "I know I can get well now. I feel better already.

EPILOGUE

Ron and Sharon liked the Cancer Center so well, they stayed the whole nine months. Both of them went through a healing reaction or "crisis." Then they slowly rebuilt their bodies back into glowing health. They then opted, however reluctantly, to return to the year 2008.

Sharon is now a Counselor for Cancer patients in her normal time zone. Ron is inventing exercise equipment for specific Cancers. Both have kept up the healing program they learned at Cancer Centers of America. They have remained good friends and see each other often. In the following years, neither ever experienced a recurrence.

AUTHORS NOTE: Ron Jones is based on an actual Cancer patient. Jones, an innovative and creative black man, died at age forty-eight while receiving "standard" medical treatment for his Gastric Cancer in a Los Angeles hospital in 2004. Sharon is fictional, based on the many women I have encountered in the eighteen years I have been speaking and writing about Cancer. Her story is typical of those I have heard.

CHAPTER 29

The Time is Now to Conquer Cancer

AFTER SPENDING EIGHTEEN years talking to people with Cancer and putting in a lot of time in the field, I am convinced that we can prevent and overcome Cancer **now.** We don't have to wait for "Advances in Medicine", new Biotech discoveries, new cutting-edge Medical treatments, or the discovery of the ever-elusive "Cure."

Progress in Cancer will come when we wake up from our fantasy-land mind set that disease can be cut, poisoned, or burned out of the body, take responsibility for our health, and do the wonderful work of self-healing and self-lumpectomy using entirely natural, supportive means.

Cancer is as much a state of the body and mind as it is a disease. We can get into that state when we encounter a huge emotional, financial or other traumatic stress, when we ingest or are exposed to way too many toxins in our working, home, medical or general environment, and /or when we neglect our health. When we indulge in self-destructive habits like smoking, drinking, drug addictions, overeating, harboring anger and resentment, and experiencing conflicted relationships for a long period of time, we jeopardize our health. A selfish lifestyle in which we may use or even hurt others in pursuit of personal gain also is a suspect, as this is an accurate description of the way Cancer cells behave.

When we are in denial about our distresses and do not talk about them, seek help, or express them in some creative way, they can be bottled up inside creating havoc. A subsequent depression, however unacknowledged, can depress our immune system that no longer can act as a "security guard" against Cancer cells. *Our cells are a mirror-reflection of our own behavior.*

In the eighteen years after my healing from Breast and Uterine Cancer on the MOTEP program, I have never had a recurrence. I am still on the MOTEP program. Mending bad relationships from my own selfish, inconsiderate behavior in the past has taken a high priority. This has proven more difficult than the exercise program I regularly follow, the low-fat diet that has me at my ideal weight, or even the regular chanting and visualization that I practice. But it has been far more rewarding than even wearing the size six apparel I now purchase. I have learned a lot about maintaining my health, especially in times of crisis and the true rewards of helping others to realize they can get well.

For example, I was awakened by a jangling phone at half-past midnight. A paramedic was loudly and emphatically telling me that he found my mother in extreme danger, cold and with low-blood pressure. He felt that my father had waited too long to call 911. He thought perhaps she had food poisoning, he wasn't sure. He was taking her to the hospital and urged me to make the trip to Reno as promptly as I could to be with her.

My mother was eighty-three at the time. She now is eighty-eight. Dad was eighty-nine. He now is ninety-four.

My mother, Amy, has been my "Stage Mother" all my life, urging me on in my creative efforts of painting, drawing, and writing. She has been my stalwart when times were tough. Just like Stephen Sprouse, the fashion designer who died at age fifty, my life has been a roller coaster of financial and emotional ups and downs.

Beginner's luck was with me when I showed my paintings and drawings on Madison Avenue in the Seventies, at age thirty-two. The eighties were also a whirlwind of success for me when I was in my forties. I became convinced that money flowed in like a river because my art was so great, etc. Going to upscale restaurants and buying designer clothes were par for the course for me and my friends whom I often treated.

However, as the eighties disappeared, so did my income. I well remember the year 1989, when sales stopped completely, as if hitting a brick wall with a loud thud! It was then, I believe, that I began my downhill journey into Cancer. The two tumors showed up in December 1990 at my regular gynecologist appointment. It had been almost two years of desperation. I had also lost a boyfriend I thought was the love of my life when he ran off and married a woman he had visited for twenty years.

Now my mother was in trouble, perhaps on her deathbed, I thought. I made arrangements to immediately fly to Reno, even moving the trip up to that very weekend when my brother became hysterical. For the first few days she was in the hospital, I talked to her over the phone every day several times, even though she could barely speak. I then boarded a plane for the trip.

In Reno, having been given a key, I was at the house to open the door when she was semi-carried in, as she could barely walk. I took care of her for the next several days, becoming *her* Mother. I shopped, cooked and stayed with her for hours at a time. I kissed her cheek. Mother came from a cold family and affection was never displayed. But I knew from my experience that love is a key ingredient in healing.

Soon she became stronger. She began walking with the aid of a walker. By the time I left, she was back on her feet. She could walk on her own! The next week she wrote that she had prepared my father's vegetable soup for him in gratitude for his immense caring. My father usually fixes his own meals. He had been with her in the hospital every day.

STRESS TAKES A TOLL

When I returned from Reno, I thought I could go back to work in my Studio as if nothing had transpired. The huge emotional stress and trauma that I had been under, however, had taken its toll. I began to have stomach problems and residual pain from past accidents throughout my body. I did not sleep soundly. I realized I was exhausted and emotionally spent.

I have become very aware of the state of my health. I am no longer in denial. I can stand up for myself against anyone. I defend myself against any attack. I also know when my body is beginning a downhill course and I feel debilitated. Here was a perfect opportunity for me to go into a downhill spiral and once more experience ill health and perhaps even a Cancer recurrence.

Instead, I acknowledged my declining health and gave myself a day off. I went out to the spa. Starting early, I did half an hour of swimming in the mineral pool. I soaked in the sulphur pools, always extremely tranquilizing for me. After lunch, I visited the clay pool and covered myself with mineral-rich "mud," found a chaise lounge and under the sunny sky, promptly fell sound asleep! When I awoke, I washed off the clay and did half an hour of water aerobics with the group in the pool. I made friends with many others also aware that they needed a day of rejuvenation. After the visit to the spa, I felt totally rejuvenated. Then, back home that night, I was able to sleep like a rock!

The next day I was back in the studio, fully recovered and able to work hard once again. The aches and pains were completely gone and I felt strong and energetic.

BECOME AWARE WHEN LIFE THREATENS TO CAUSE DISEASE

I fully believe that when we become aware that our life-condition is slipping downhill, that we can ourselves practice "early detection" and avoid slipping further into the disease called Cancer. If we do break down into this state, I believe we can reverse it and retrieve our precious health by a process of slow but sure internal cleansing and healing, not dependant on drugs, surgery, or radiation. I have written this book to give hope, not "false hope" but real hope to anyone who fears or is diagnosed with any type of Cancer. It is my belief you can prevent Cancer. You can get well from any Cancer. And you can stay well.

Make the effort to change your life, to acquire the new habits that will lead you to the high road to health and well-being. Go on the MOTEP program I have outlined in this book. You will be extremely happy you did. And your body will rejoice!

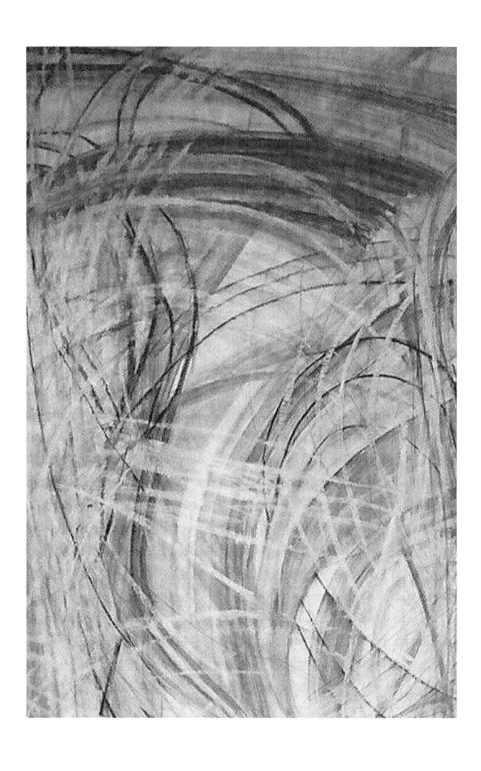

Foods with Laetrile—Vitamin B-17

FORTY-ONE FOODS CONTAINING LAETRILE
(Vitamin B-17)

Used throughout history to kill Cancer
cells and prevent Cancer.
(*Ernest Krebs*)

1. Apple seeds

2. Alfalfa sprouts

3. Apricot kernels
   (two-four per day only)

4. Bamboo shoots

5. Barley

6. Beet tops

7. Bitter almond

8. Blackberries

9. Boysenberries

10. Brewer's yeast

11. Brown rice

12. Buckwheat

13. Cashews

14. Cherry kernels

15. Cranberries

16. Currants

17. Fava beans

18. Flax seeds

19. Filberts

20. Garbanzo beans

21. Gooseberries

22. Huckleberries

23. Lentils

24. Lima beans

25. Linseed Meal

26. Loganberries

27. Macadamia nuts

28. Millet

29. Millet seed

30. Peach kernels

31. Pecans

32. Plum kernels

33. Quince

34. Raspberries

35. Sorghum Can Syrup

36. Spinach

37. Sprouts (alfalfa, lentil, mung bean, buckwheat, garbanzo)

38. Strawberries

39. Walnuts

40. Watercress

41. Yams

Some Healthy Cookbooks

1. Arnot, Bob *The Breast Cancer Prevention Diet*, New York, Little Brown & Co. 1999.

2. Mayhew, Debra *The Soup Bible*, New York, Barnes and Noble, 2004.

3. Daley, Rosie and Weil, Andrew, M.D. *The Healthy Kitchen*, New York, Alfred Knopf, 2003.

4. Madison, Deborah, *Vegetarian Cooking for Everyone*, New York, Broadway Books, 1997.

5. Kordich, Jay, *The Juiceman's Power of Juicing*, New York, Warner Books, 1993.

6. Katzan, Molly, *New Classics—350 Recipes for Homestyle Favorites and Everyday Feasts,* New York, Clarkson Potter, 2001.

7. Underkoffler, Renee Loux, *Living Cuisine—The Art and Spirit of Raw Foods*, New York, Avery/ Penguin, 2003.

8. Shurtleff, William and Aoyagi, Akiko, *The Book of Tofu*, Berkeley, Ca. Ten Speed Press, 2001.

9. Dragonwagon, Crescent, *Passionate Vegetarian*, New York, Workman, 2002.

10. Petrovna, Tanya, *Native Foods Restaurant Cookbook*, Boston, Shambhala, 2003.

11. Jones, Jeanne, *Canyon Ranch Cooking, Bringing the Sea Home*, New York, HarperCollins, 1998.

12. Hendricks, Judith Ryan, *Bread Alone*, New York, William Morrow, 2001.

13. Chang, Irving B., Kutscher, Helene W.and Austin, *An Encyclopedia of Chinese Food and Cooking*, Crown, 1970.

14. Greenberg, Patricia, *The Whole Soy Cookbook*, New York, Three Rivers Press, 1998.

Danger of Biopsies

RALPH MOSS REPORTS on a Clinical Trial done for a paper on the safety of biopsies done at John Wayne Cancer Institute in Santa Monica, California. The needle and core biopsies were examined to see if they actually resulted in the spread of Cancer, because the encapsulated tumor holds Cancer cells like an eggshell that protects its contents and encloses it. Once poked into mechanically, it was feared, the Cancer cells would be released and spread, perhaps unchecked throughout the body.

The author of the study was Nora M. Hanson, M.D., Chief Surgical Resident at the University of Chicago, before coming to Santa Monica, California, to be Assistant Director of the Joyce Eisenberg Keefer Breast Center.

She questioned this standard, routine procedure for obtaining specimens to analyze for Cancer cells. Enrolled in the study were 683 women with Breast Cancer. Half had been biosied with a needle—either a fine needle aspiration or a large-guage needle core biopsy. The other half had their whole tumor excised, (excisional biopsy or lumpectomy).

The study found that women who had either kind of needle biopsy were fifty percent more likely to have Cancer in their sentinal lymph nodes than women who underwent the surgical removal of the whole tumor.

"The implications of this study are vast, since patients who are found to have Cancer in their lymph nodes are automatically classified at a higher stage, Ralph Moss writes.

Genes are Not Destiny

"UPENDING THE PREVAILING genetic theory, a team of scientists at Purdue University has discovered a mechanism in plants that allows them to correct defective genes from their parents by tapping into an ancestral data bank of healthy genetic material," Karen Kaplan reports in the *Los Angeles Times.*

The study upturns the widely embraced laws of Mendelian genetics, dating back to the mid-1800s, that holds that plants and animals inherit only two copies of a gene—one from each parent. If both copies were defective, a plant would have no ability to correct the error.

The Purdue scientists happened upon their discovery accidentally. They were intending to study a deformed version of the Arabidopsis plant that produced flowers fused into tight balls because of two defective copies of a gene dubbed "hot-head."

Breeding these Hot-Heads should have resulted in deformed offspring, but scientists were startled to see that ten percent were normal flowers. Genes may have modified in the DNA, or by the RNA, a close cousin.

This research also questions the testing for BRCA 1 and BRCA2 gene mutations to frighten women into accepting "prophylactic" mastectomies for their healthy breasts. *Genes are not destiny*.

The way we take care of our body, mind, and spirit, is what counts in the prevention of Cancer. Although there is no money in it, breast amputations will, I predict, will be replaced by self-care and self-healing methods that are natural and safe. Mastectomies will become a horrendous oddity of the past, shocking future generations who read about them.

Further Reading

1. Arnot, Bob and Jim Arnosky, *The Breast Cancer Prevention Diet*. New York, Little Brown & Co. 1999.

2. Null, Gary, *Power Aging: The Revolutionary Program to Control Symptoms of Aging Naturally*. New York, American Library, 2003. Also, any health books by Gary Null.

3. Anderson, Norman B. Ph.D. with Elizabeth Anderson, *Emotional Longevity–What Really Determines How Long You Live*. New York, Penguin, 2003.

4. Goldberg, Burton, *Cancer Diagnosis–What To Do Next*. Berkeley, Ca. Ten Speed Press, 2000.

5. Frahm, Anne and David J. Frahm, *Cancer Battle Plan–Six Strategies for Beating Cancer from a Recovered, Hopeless Case*, New York, Jeremy Tarcher/ Putnam, 1998.

6. Hirshberg, Caryle and Marc Ian Barasch, *Remarkable Recovery*. Riverhead Books, 1955. Republished Garden City, N.Y. Square One Publishers, 2004.

7. Temoshek, Lydia, Ph.D. and Dreher, Henry, *The Type C Connection: The Behavioral Links To Your Health*. New York, Random House, 1992.

8. Keuneke, Robin, *Total Breast Health: Power Foods for Protection and Wellness*. New York, Kensington Books, 1998.

9. Daniel, Rosy, with Ellis, Rachel, *The Cancer Prevention Book: A Complete Mind/Body Approach to Stopping Cancer Before it Starts*. Berkeley, Ca. Hunter House, 1998.

10. Health Experts at The Doctors' Prescription for Healthy Living Magazine, *Natural Cancer Cures*, Topanga, Ca. Freedom Press, 2008.

11. Calbom, Cherie M.S., Calbom, John and Manaffey, Michael, *The Complete Cancer Cleanse*, Nashville, Tennessee, Thomas Nelson, Inc., 2006.

12. Quillan, Patrick, *Beating Cancer with Nutrition*, Carlsbad, Ca. Nutrition Times Press, Revised 2005.

13. LeShan, Lawrence, Ph.D., *Cancer as a Turning Point*, New York, Plume Books, Revised 1994.

Index

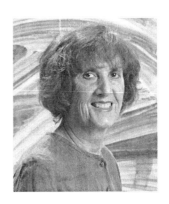

About the Author

SUSAN MOSS has been saving lives since she was a teenage life-guard in Reno, Nevada. In 1967, along with Dr. James B. Nichols, she started a Suicide Prevention Hotline at the University of Nevada, which is still in operation today.

Her book, *Keep Your Breasts! Preventing Breast Cancer the Natural Way* is an International Best-Seller—published in three languages and in its sixth printing—has been on the shelf of major bookstores for fifteen years.

An Artist with five hundred collectors including three major Museums, Susan Moss has spent her life thinking creatively. When she was diagnosed with Breast and Uterine Cancer in December 1990, she thought outside the box and created an all-natural health program to heal herself naturally. She has been healthy and free of Cancer for eighteen years. Thousands of men and women have benefited from her hard-won knowledge.